'You ask me what were the secret forces which sustained me during my long fasts. Well, it was my unshakable faith in God, my simple and frugal life style, and the Aloe whose benefits I discovered upon my arrival in South Africa at the end of the 19th century.'

Mahatma Gandhi

In a letter to his biographer Romain Rolland

TITLE
THE ESSENTIAL ALOE VERA
THE ACTIONS AND THE EVIDENCE

AUTHOR
Dr. Peter Atherton

Published by Mill Enterprises, Park Farm, Gayhurst, Newport Pagnell MK16 8LG. UK

To Alison

A patient who changed my practice.

1st Edition 1996
2nd Edition 1997

Printed by: Northward Press, 18 Ballmoor, Buckingham Industrial Park
Buckingham MK18 1RT

Published by: Mill Enterprises

Global Literary Agents and Distributors - Aloe World Limited
e-mail: aloeworldlimited@aol.com

ISBN 0-9540896-0-X

Contents

AUTHOR'S NOTE

This handbook is designed for educational purposes only and does not endorse any particular brand or type of Aloe Vera products.

Dr Atherton regrets that he is unable to directly enter into any correspondence regarding his opinion on the use of Aloe Vera in particular case histories.

Acknowledgements

I would like to thank my wife, Ellen, for suffering with me during our holiday in which I transferred my thoughts to paper and for being my sounding board.

My thanks also to good friend, Glenda Goodwin, for typing out the original manuscript. I commend her for her patience in making the many changes and corrections.

My eternal thanks to Alison whose personal experience with Aloe Vera led to a change in my practice of medicine after twenty-five years of a purely conventional approach.

I have also received huge help from Tamsin Wright-Carpenter in the compilation of the references and from Pam Richardson in collating the Anthraquinone Section. Also, thanks to Nick Hutchins for his invaluable advice.

Finally, I would like to thank Forever Living Products (UK) Ltd., for the use of their photographs of Aloe Vera plants.

INTRODUCTION

"Aloe, what? yes, I think that I've heard of it. That stuff they put in cosmetics."

This was part of a conversation that took place just over three years ago with a patient of mine. She was the mother of a little boy with eczema, whose problem had apparently 'miraculously' cleared up completely after applying a cream containing Aloe Vera with bee propolis. In case you don't know, as I didn't at the time, bee propolis is obtained from the lining of bee hives and is the substance responsible for keeping the hive sterile. It is known to possess powerful antimicrobial properties which make the inside of a beehive more sterile than an operating theatre. Bees make propolis by collecting resins from trees such as pines and poplars, which they then mix with their own enzymes to create the sticky substance called propolis or bee glue.

Since then I have been fortunate to meet with Dr William Davey who, amongst other things holds a Royal Charter as Honorary Homeopathic Physician to Her Majesty The Queen. He started life as a chest physician but he has also been involved in research. A main part of that research has been into bee propolis and his findings are shortly to be published as a thesis. In it he will demonstrate the active ingredient in propolis which is a most powerful antimicrobial agent, capable of even killing mycobacterium tuberculosis. He has also shown that the propolis itself is more active as a whole than the pure extract. This idea of synergy in plant ingredients is a theme that I will be dwelling on later in the book, as I believe in the truth of an Ayruvedic text from India:

"Extracting drugs from a part of a plant is taking out the intelligence and throwing away the wisdom".

The conversation with that mother was not only to change my attitude to Aloe Vera, but also to herbal, nutritional, and complementary medicine in general. In fact, it would totally change my approach to the practice of medicine, and change my life.

At the time, I confess I was rather irritated by the mother's remarks and certainly very sceptical as she went on to tell me that I must try the cream because it had succeeded where all my moisturisers and steroid creams had failed. Eczema, of course, is known to naturally wax and wane, so it had to be coincidental, didn't it?

Up to then I had been a General Practitioner for twenty-five years and a strictly conventional one at that. I left it to my partners to indulge in acupuncture, homoeopathy, applied kinesiology and nutritional medicine.

As this patient was also a friend, it was not long before we met again and inevitably the subject of Aloe Vera came up. But now I was invited to drink the stuff as well as rub it on! The more uses she mentioned, the more I switched off and the more sceptical I became. However, I knew she wouldn't go away so I promised that I would read the company literature that she had given me on the previous occasion.

The company was biased, as I expected it to be, but there was something about this herb's history that caught my interest. There were references to Alexander the Great, Cleopatra and Nefertiti, no doubt a mythical association, but it prompted me to go as far as asking the secretary of my local post-graduate medical centre to dig out anything she could find on Aloe Vera.

She came up with forty papers from around the world. Although some were from fairly dubious sources, with only one exception they all had something very positive to say about Aloe Vera. Such a high incidence of enthusiasm is very unusual in medical papers and it is also rare to find such a consensus.

One paper in particular, from the Acne Research Institute of California, published in the Journal of Dermatological Surgery on post dermabrasion wound healing, was to commit me to using Aloe Vera myself as well as in my practice. There were two reasons that this paper fired my imagination: first, my favourite aspect of general practice is dermatology and second, the content of the paper was very interesting. Dermabrasion is a very aggressive way of treating badly scarred skin following the ravages of facial acne, by literally shaving off the epidermis, or skin surface, leaving the raw area of the dermis to heal and regenerate a smoother epidermal layer. This is fine if all goes well and the healing is swift and without any infection. But it is obviously risky and, in the worst case, can lead to a situation which is more disfiguring than before.

British medicine is generally more conservative than that in the USA, so dermabrasion is only rarely performed here. However, during this experiment in California, they added Aloe Vera gel to their standard post-operative dressing and applied it to one side of the face in several patients, leaving the other side with just their standard mixture. They found that the side with the Aloe Vera gel consistently healed seventy-two hours faster than the one without Aloe Vera gel. This was remarkable because the healing was some 25-30 per cent faster. The paper ended by stating: "The cause of the accelerated healing is not known". That did it. I had to know more about this unusual plant. Three years later, I am still very excited about its potential and I am still learning.

As a direct consequence of using Aloe Vera myself, in my family and in my practice, I made the decision to try and research its medicinal qualities in depth. Shortly after a wonderful opportunity appeared. By chance, I found out that any general practitioner could apply for prolonged study leave for up to a year, subsidised by the National Health Service. All the candidate had to do, with the endorsement of their regional post graduate Dean and two referees, was to make a case for a research project that would both promote the doctor's professional growth and benefit National Health Service patients. I never for a minute thought that my application would be successful but I had a stroke of luck - always necessary with most ventures. When I telephoned the Department of Health to check that my application had been received, I was informed by a young man who was responsible for "rubber stamping" the document that he had only been in the job for a week and was not too familiar with the process! Well, I enlightened him on the need for a speedy assessment in order to arrange locums etc. What followed was a very sympathetic conversation about his difficulties in joining a new department. Having once been a civil servant myself I understood his problems, and so before I had put the phone down, the business had been resolved and I was planning my sabbatical year!

In another fortunate encounter with the Clinical Professor of Dermatology at Oxford, it was suggested that I could also apply for a visiting research fellowship at Green college, Oxford and carry out my work in the Department of Dermatology and work with the Oxford Institute of Wound Healing. I would have a desk in the visitors room which I would share, amongst others, with Dr. Gerry Bodeker, Chairman of the Global Initiative for Traditional Systems of Health - GIFTS of health as it is commonly known.

I was granted my fellowship and the association with these talented people was to prove most enjoyable and fruitful.

At the time of writing my fellowship year is sadly coming to an end but I have now completed my major task. This was to seek out and evaluate the world-wide literature written on all aspects of Aloe Vera.

I hope to publish my findings in conjunction with Dr. Tom Reynolds, Senior Lecturer at the Jodrell Laboratory, Royal Botanic Gardens, Kew, as an updated review in an academic journal. The purpose of this second edition of "The Essential Aloe Vera" is to provide the evidence that might persuade my colleagues, and other health professionals and interested people, of the place of Aloe Vera in a system of integrated medicine, where the best of conventional or allopathic medicine can be combined with the best of natural or complementary medicine; all evidence based of course.

Having read this short book, I hope that more people, particularly those involved in the provision of health care, will understand the properties and uses of Aloe Vera, so that they can see for themselves the benefits to be obtained, especially in areas where conventional medicine has little or nothing to offer. I am certainly not discouraging the acceptance of the conventional approach, however, I do believe Aloe Vera has a complementary role to play in the management of several conditions, but it is not just for the sick. Healthy people can benefit tremendously from its superb qualities, all of which will be discussed later.

At first, I was going to write a separate book on my research findings but I have decided to expand the original book and combine it with much more science and many more references. Because I would like to appeal to a wider audience, not just those scientifically orientated, I have highlighted the areas of the more technical data so that the book can be read without reference to these at all. However, if the reader would like to investigate any or all of the more biological or biochemical aspects, they are immediately available.

As there are too many references to number the text, I have divided the references into sections relating to a particular aspect of the plant and, where I consider a reference to be particularly important, I have highlighted it in bold type. A commentary on each section will be given in Part II.

PART I

THE HISTORY

As I said in the introduction, it was the history of Aloe Vera that first aroused my fascination with the plant, for it has truly stood the test of time and has been associated with some remarkable people.

The name Aloe Vera, or true Aloe, is probably derived from the Arabic word 'ALLOEH', Syrian 'ALWAI' or Hebrew 'HALAL' meaning a 'shining bitter substance'. Hence the old laxative remedy 'bitter Aloes', still listed in the US Pharmacopea today.

The German Egyptologist, George Ebers (1837-1898) bought an ancient papyrus, now called the Ebers Papyrus, dating from the reign of the Pharoah Amen-Hotep in 1552 BC. This ancient medical treatise listing the use of plant materials as cosmetics and drugs, including Aloes, was found between the knees of a mummy excavated near Thebes in 1858. This papyrus demonstrated the use of Aloe Vera during the preceding 2,000 years and listed twelve different formulae for Aloe Vera preparations.

Over the centuries, there have been many references to Aloe Vera, in many different cultures, from the Ancient Greeks and Romans to Babylonian, Indian and Chinese peoples. Important thinkers such as Celsius from the time of Jesus Christ, through to the Roman physician, Pliny the Elder and the Greek Dioscorides all supported the therapeutic importance of Aloe Vera. Galen, the father of modern medicine, who was the first doctor to describe how the heart and circulation worked, is known to have used it.

The first reference to Aloe Vera in English was made in AD 1655 in a translation from Dioscorides by John Goodyear. Dioscorides wrote that this bitter tasting strongly scented liquid had "the power of binding or procuring sleep, of drying, of thickening bodies, and loosening of ye belly and of cleansing of ye stomach". In addition "it stops ye spitting of blood and it cleanseth ye icterus (liver)" and finally, "it properly healeth exulterated genitalls". Dioscorides wrote *De Materia Medica* from which this was translated in AD70-90. In this treatise he catalogued and described more than 600 plants and plant principles. Dioscorides certainly got it right when it came to treating genital lesions as a most recent paper by Dr T A Syed et al, published last year, showed that a topical 0.5% Aloe Vera extract in a randomised double blind trial, significantly healed the lesions of genital herpes faster than a control, and prevented recurrence.

Traders first brought Aloe to London in 1693 and, by 1843, 4,227 gourds were being imported each year.

Although physicians had prescribed Aloe for more than 2,000 years, it was not until 1851 that T & H. Smith of Edinburgh discovered Aloin, which they believed in small doses acted as a tonic assisting digestion and exerting a special influence on the liver. In larger doses it became a strong laxative. Throughout the 18th and 19th centuries Aloe remained one of the more popular prescribed and over the counter medicines.

The presence or absence of Aloin in modern Aloe Vera products is a controversial issue. Some companies filter it out, whereas others leave a little in, so I will look at this closely in the section on Anthraquinones, in which chemical group it falls.

There are also many fables and myths surrounding Aloe Vera's history. For example, that the Egyptian queens, Cleopatra and Nefertiti were thought to have used Aloe as part of their beauty regimes but, unfortunately, this is not genuinely documented and is probably wishful thinking.

Alexander the Great, after conquering Persia in 333 BC, was said to have been persuaded by his mentor Aristotle, to capture the island of Socotra in the Indian Ocean. This battle was fought in order to secure the island's famed Aloe supplies that were needed to treat Alexander's wounded soldiers. I did not believe this to be true at first, as Alexander travelled home by land! However, I have subsequently learnt that he sent one of his generals home by sea. Could he have been the victor of Socotra?

Another popular myth is that Aloe Vera is referred to in the Bible. In fact, it is lignin Aloe that is mentioned there five times, but not Aloe Vera. The most famous passage comes from St. John's Gospel: "And there came also, Nicodemus, which at the first came to Jesus by night, and brought a mixture of myrrh, and aloes, about a hundred pounds weight ..." Lignin Aloe is a tree with a scented bark which was used to make incense as well as for the preservation and embalming of the dead.

The true Aloe has been endowed with such marvellous properties that, over the years and in the different areas of the world, the Aloe has been given many wonderful names:

Burn plant	Dietary plant
Healing plant	Heaven's blessing
Medicine plant	Plant of life
Potted physician	Wonder plant
Wand of heaven	First aid plant
Silent Healer	Single Bible

THE PLANT AND ITS STRUCTURE

In order to understand Aloe Vera's ability to act as a medicinal herb one must have some knowledge of its general structure and the contents of the leaves. So, first let us look at it from a botanical point of view and see where it fits into the plant kingdom.

Description

Aloe Vera is a succulent belonging to the lily family (Liliacae). In this family there are about 3,700 species of flowering plants, but also included are garlic, onion and asparagus of which the former is also accredited medicinal properties. Aloe Vera itself, forms part of a subspecies (the Aloinae) of which there are at least 200 to 300 types. No one seems to know exactly how many there are.

Most species are non-toxic but there are about 15 poisonous ones containing a deadly hemlock-like substance - the method chosen by Socrates to commit suicide.

Of the true Aloes there are probably only four or five with documented medicinal benefits. These are:

1. Aloe Barbadensis Miller sometimes called: Aloe Linne or Aloe Vulgaris or the Curacao Aloe.

2. Aloe Perryi Baker, the Socotrine Aloe or Zanzibar Aloe

3. Aloe Ferox often called Cape Aloe.

4. The last two and least popular are Aloe Arborescens and Aloe Saponaria which are mainly used in Japan.

Of all of these, Aloe Barbadensis Miller is the most potent and is the one generally used in commercial preparations in the UK and USA.

It is really the only species that should be called Aloe Vera and this name should really be reserved exclusively for the Barbadensis Miller variety. This is because it was first referred to by this name in a South African publication "Flora Indira" by N L Burman in 1768. This description preceded the publication of Miller's dictionary by at least ten days! This gives it priority.

The species is indigenous to Africa, but these plants have become widely distributed both in the Near and Far East as well as the West Indies (Aloe Vera arrived on the Caribbean island of Barbados in about 1650), and the drier parts of Europe such as Spain.

Aloe Vera thrives in warm, rather arid areas. Its one great enemy is frost, so it grows well as a pot plant in the home, but not outside. If you have one growing on your window-sill, when you next get a bite, a sting or a burn, just cut off a leaf and squeeze the gel out on to the painful area and rub it in. Feel the 'First Aid Plant' at work!

The Structure

The plant takes four to five years to reach maturity when its leaves, which grow from a short stem, are about 60 cm (2 feet) in length and about 8-10 cm (3-4 inches) wide at the base. The leaves taper to a point and possess soft marginal spines. If the stem is cut transversely the leaves can be seen to be growing in a rosette pattern.

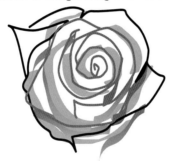

From the middle of the mass of dark-green leaves, the flower stem develops reaching about 90 cm (3 feet) in length and has long, rather tubular yellow flowers. At the base of the mother plant little 'suckers', or 'pups', grow which are easily separated to make new cuttings. The plant can also reproduce by cross fertilisation. In the wild the method of pollination is often by humming birds.

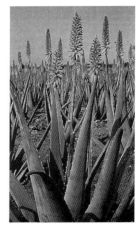

Aloe Vera, being a perennial, has the life span of about twelve years, but the leaves are usually harvested at about three to four years of age. When the outer leaves are harvested, possibly up to three times a year, the plant is able to 'seal' itself against water loss. This protective habit is peculiar to succulents. Within a few seconds of the wound being inflicted it films over and during the next few minutes a rubber-like protective coating stops further loss of sap, so the stem does not become dessicated and continues to live. In a short time the wound heals completely. No wonder it's called the Wand of Heaven!

Inside the Leaf

The structure of the Aloe leaf (seen below in cross-section) shows the outer-rind about fifteen cell layers thick. This is dark-green in colour and has a hard, waxy surface. The hardness is due to the large amounts of calcium and magnesium present in it. The greenness comes from chlorophyll which uses sunlight, carbon dioxide and water to manufacture the Aloe Vera gel. Below the rind are vascular bundles, or tubes, of xylem and phloem. The xylem transports water and minerals from the roots upwards into the leaves, providing ingredients for the manufacturing process.

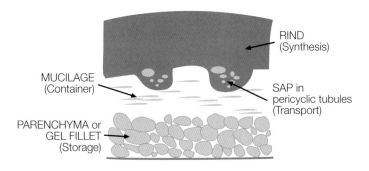

The phloem transports the synthesised materials down to the roots and other parts of the leaf. Small pericyclic tubules connect these, and larger tubules running lengthwise down the leaf take nourishment to the young 'pups'. Next comes a mucilage layer of long, chain polysaccharides, (the relevance of which will be discussed later), forming a container to hold the inner parenchyma or gel. It also maintains the sterility of the inner gel.

When a leaf is cut and held up, sap will quickly drain out of the larger tubules and, if this were used on its own, it would provide a stunning laxative, because it is composed largely of anthraquinones which we will look at in the next section.

The leaf and its contents

In analysing the contents of the leaf, I shall be looking at the three essential ingredients:

- the sap
- the mucilage
- the parenchymatous gel.

There are over seventy-five known ingredients in the Aloe Vera leaf, divided into eight distinct categories, and I suspect that there are still others to be discovered. However, there is some confusion over the exact content of some of the fractions, so I will present a consensus opinion, gleaned from a recent literature review. The solid fraction only forms some 0.5 - 1.5% of the plant so this is a relatively small amount. Its average pH value is 4.55. In the next chapter we will look at how and where these ingredients work.

Lignin

A cellulose based substance found in the gel with no known specific medicinal properties, but it is thought to provide the property of penetration of the human skin in Aloe preparations that contain it.

Saponins

Glycosides are thought to comprise about 3 per cent of Aloe Vera gel. They are soapy substances capable of cleansing, and with antiseptic properties.

Anthraquinones and Derivatives

There are twelve of these in the complex listed below:

Aloin	Barbaloin
Isobarbaloin	Anthranol
Anthracene	Aloetic acid
Emodin	Aloe Emodin
Ester of Cinnamonic acid	Ethereal oil
Chrysophanic acid	Resistannol

These compounds are found in the sap alone. Traditionally they are known as laxatives, and in high concentration on their own, they can be toxic, but within the complex environment of the Aloe Vera plant they are not. They are excellent analgesics, or pain killers, and they also possess powerful antibacterial, antifungal and virucidal activity.

In order to obtain the painkilling benefit as well as the ability to enhance absorption from the gut, some sap containing anthraquinones should be present in any Aloe drink. When present it is obvious, as anthraquinones impart a bitter taste and add to the yellow or orange colour of the gel/sap mixture. Aloin in high concentration is toxic to fibroblasts so too much Aloin in topical products would kill these cells in the dermis and retard healing by lessening fibre production. However, they do have some beneficial skin effects which will be described later.

Chemistry of Anthraquinones

The main anthraquinone found in the sap, latex or resin in Aloe Vera is Barbaloin which is synonymous with Aloin. There are also the derivatives which are anthrones and chromones. These form the phenolic fraction of the sap.

Barbaloin is an
anthrone - c - glycoside

13

After ingestion Aloin is converted by bacterial action in the large bowel to Aloe-emodin-9-anthrone. This is the active ingredient which causes an increase in water content of the large intestine by inhibiting electrolyte absorption and stimulating electrolyte secretion. It may also stimulate peristalsis.

Minerals

Calcium	Magnesium
Sodium	Zinc
Iron	Manganese
Potassium	Copper
Chromium	

There are about thirty vitamins, minerals and trace elements which are essential for good health and should be consumed on a regular basis. Many of them work together and depend on others in order to function properly. I have listed the more important properties and functions below.

Calcium

Primarily has a structural role in bones and teeth but it is also essential for cellular structure and nerve transmission. It needs a balance of phosphorous and magnesium to work effectively and Vitamin D is required for its absorption.

Manganese

This is a component of many enzymes and is necessary for the activation of other enzymes. These substances are complex proteins which act as biochemical catalysts thereby speeding up the route of clinical reaction in the plant.

Sodium

This is a very important mineral, responsible for preventing body fluids from becoming too acid or too alkaline. It is also involved in the electrical conductivity in muscles and nerves as well as the uptake of nutrients by individual cells.

Copper

Also a component of a number of enzymes and involved in enabling iron to operate as an oxygen carrier in red blood cells.

Magnesium

This is intimately involved in calcium metabolism during the formation of bone and is needed by nerves and muscle membranes to allow them to conduct electrical impulses.

Potassium

Like sodium, this is involved in the acid-base balance in the body and also electrical conductivity in muscles and nerves.

Zinc

Is involved in major metabolic pathways contributing to the metabolism of proteins, carbohydrates (sugars) and fats. An inadequate intake would have an adverse effect on any tissue that dies and is renewed rapidly such as skin, gut lining or the immune system. Recent studies have shown that the desperate condition of schizophrenia may be associated with zinc deficiency.

Chromium

This is necessary for the proper function of insulin, which in turn controls blood sugar levels, so all diabetics require a good intake of chromium.

Iron

It is the "haem" part of haemoglobin in red blood cells which enables the transport of oxygen around the body as oxyhaemoglobin. Iron deficiency anaemia is very common in those with poor nutrition and in any case where there is depletion through chronic blood loss e.g. excessive menstruation.

The Vitamins

Vitamin Bl	Vitamin B12	Folic Acid
Vitamin B2	Vitamin C	(Vitamin C)*
Vitamin B6	Beta Carotene (Vitamin A)	(Vitamin E)'
Choline	Niacinamide (Niacin)	

*Extra vitamins are often added to the natural ones in the plant extract as they form part of the stabilisation process which ensures that the commercial product remains as near to the natural juice as possible, and also acts as a preservative.

Vitamins A, C and E

These are the important antioxidant vitamins, which are essential to fight the dangerous free radicals. They influence the immune system and Vitamin C, particularly, assists in wound healing whereas Vitamin A is required to maintain normal and night vision.

Free radicals are constantly being formed by normal body processes, but they are also produced by any form of combustion such as smoking, exhaust fumes, radiation and even the burning of food, such as on a barbecue or in a frying pan. They will try to oxidise tissues and cause great damage triggering everything from cancers to cataracts, arterial disease and premature ageing. Look what oxygen does to metal when it oxidises it. It produces rust and eventually destroys it - powerful stuff.

These oxidising free radicals must be neutralised by the antioxidants, (the main ones are Vitamins A, C and E), but also by the mineral selenium and micro-nutrients called bioflavonoids, so I doubt whether you can have too many antioxidants in your diet.

The B Vitamins, including Choline

These are associated with the production of energy and with amino acid metabolism, so associated with developing muscle mass.

Vitamin B 12

This is one of the few plant sources of this essential vitamin needed for making red blood cells, and deficiency will lead to anaemia.

Folic Acid

Is very important in the development of blood cells as deficiency will cause anaemia.

Amino Acids

The human body requires twenty-two amino acids for good health and all but eight can be made in the body. The others, called essential amino acids, have to be taken in as food and together they form the building blocks of proteins from which we manufacture and repair muscle, etc.

I will not list all the amino acids but suffice to say that Aloe Vera provides twenty of the twenty-two required and seven of the eight essential ones. The missing amino acid is tryptophan, although Bill Coates, an American pharmacist and Aloe expert, claims it has this one too. I am not so sure, but to get seven out of eight has to be pretty good anyway.

Enzymes

Many enzymes have been identified in Aloe Vera. Some of the most important include:

Peroxidase	Cellulase
Aliiase	Carboxypeptidase
Catalase	Amylase
Lipase	Alkaline Phosphatase

These enzymes help to break down food and therefore aid digestion. Some break down starch and sugars, for example, amylase, while others catalyse reactions to break down fats, for example, lipase. The nutrients in our food therefore, can be more efficiently absorbed.

Sugars

Aloe Vera contains both monosaccharides such as glucose and fructose and polysaccharides of which perhaps the most important are the polysaccharides. A most significant polysaccharide has been isolated by Carrington Laboratories in the USA under the trade name 'Carrisyn'. This demands special attention in relation to the immune system and will be discussed in a later chapter.

This group of polysaccharides has been called gluco-mannans or polymannose because molecules of mannose are linked to molecules of glucose but there are a few more of the mannose molecules. They vary in size tremendously from a few hundred daltons (the unit of measurement) to four million daltons and are very special sugars because of their mode of absorption from the gut. Most sugars are broken down by enzymes, absorbed piecemeal and are then reconstituted, but the long chain gluco-mannans are absorbed whole by certain cells lining the digestive tract. This action is called pinocytosis, which results in these sugars entering the blood stream in their original form.

Different members of these compounds are thought to improve arthritis, hypertension and indigestion as well as lower cholesterol, improve liver function and promote the healing of bone by increasing uptake of calcium and phosphate. In a concentrated form they have been shown to help the inflammatory bowel conditions of Crohn's disease and ulcerative colitis.

The Acemannan Story

Acemannan is a ß - (1,4) - linked acetylated mannan. It possesses three pharmacological actions:

a) primary anti-viral activity
b) secondary immunomodulating activity
c) tertiary activity in reducing opportunistic infections

It also acts synergistically with other drugs such as Azidothymide (AZT) and Acyclovir. These effects have been used in the treatment of an onchogenic retrovirus, the feline leukaemia virus, which causes a multi-syndrome disease in infected cats and has been recognised as an animal model for human immunodeficiency virus infection.

In vitro acemannan has been shown to enhance the capacity of cytotoxic 'T' lymphocytes by almost 50%. It has also been seen to activate macrophages (chicken) to produce nitric oxide. Nitric oxide acts as cytotoxic and cytostatic effector in killing tumour cells and intracellular parasites. Drugs such as Interferon can also induce nitric oxide production by macrophages. Nitric oxide may be an important factor in mediating immune regulation and host defences in mammalian and avian species. The stimulation of macrophages has been found in rats to accelerate wound healing.

At the time of writing Carrington laboratories acemannan product "Carrisyn" has reached the final stage of trials and tests before receiving a licence from the FDA for human use in the treatment of AIDS.

Sterols

These plant steroids are important anti-inflammatory agents, the four main ones being:

        Cholesterol   Campesterol
        ß Sitosterol   Lupeol

Lupeol also acts as an antiseptic and analgesic agent. Finally, Aloe Vera does contain some salicylic acid, an aspirin-like compound which together with lupeol provide some of its pain-killing properties. Other small molecules found in the solid fraction are plant hormones known as gibberellins and auxins.

WHERE DOES ALOE VERA WORK?

After reading many books, articles and papers on Aloe Vera in my quest for knowledge about this xerophyte (a plant capable of living in arid regions), I soon formed the opinion that it only seemed to work in two distinct areas.

First it became obvious that it had an effect on surfaces and membranes rather than solid organs and, secondly, on conditions that resulted from a disordered immune system. I would like to emphasise this point to deter some people from making extravagant claims about its effects in other unrelated areas and thereby giving it an ill-deserved reputation as a cure-all.

No wonder people with skin conditions and bowel conditions, asthma, as well as genital problems claim benefit from Aloe Vera for they are anatomically related, in that they are all problems affecting epithelial tissues. An epithelium is an anatomical term which is defined as a layer of cells lining the surface of the body, or a cavity that communicates with it. The skin is the largest epithelial surface and is in fact the largest organ of the body. It changes when it grows hair in the scalp but is very much still an epithelium as it is when it grows nails. When it enters the mouth the epithelium changes to become a mucous membrane as its function has changed and it does not need to preserve the body's water as normal skin does.

It continues to change as it passes through the oesophagus (gullet), stomach, the small bowel, the large bowel and finally at the anus it becomes skin again. The epithelial surface lines the nose and sinuses, trachea (wind pipe) and bronchial tubes in the lungs and it also lines the genital tract.

One of the commonest criticisms that I hear from my colleagues is that 'one substance can't possibly treat all those different conditions'. Well, of course, Aloe Vera gel is not just one substance. It is a complex interacting mixture as we've seen, containing over seventy-five ingredients, and all such conditions that benefit from Aloe Vera are linked by this common anatomical thread - the epithelium.

I could write a book solely based on anecdotal evidence about Aloe Vera but I shall only cite those events that have occurred either to me personally, my family or my patients, that is, events that I have experienced or seen with my own eyes.

Skin

Depending on its site, for damaged epithelium to receive the benefits of Aloe Vera it can be taken orally - for example, to treat indigestion or heartburn from a hiatus hernia. But as well as being ingested, it can be applied topically as in the case of skin damaged through eczema. With topical applications to the skin and scalp, general dermatological principles must still be followed, If the skin is dry then it must be moisturised, using an emollient or greasy base and, to the contrary, if the skin is oily a non-greasy base must be used. Lotions are best used in hairy areas and dressings are generally needed where skin is ulcerated.

On a personal note, to exemplify Aloe Vera's effect on chronically inflamed membranes, I discovered to my absolute joy that after taking it daily for about two weeks, my nasal catarrh, the legacy of smoking twenty cigarettes a day between 18-41 years of age, disappeared. This, of course, made breathing easier, my sense of taste improved and my tendency to snoring was removed.

The Anti-inflammatory Effect

Inflammation is the response of tissues to injury and is designed to bring cells of the immune system to the site of damage. It is a three stage reaction:

1) increased blood supply to the region
2) increase capillary permeability
3) emigration of cells out of the blood vessels into the tissues

This activity is mediated by various systems such as complement, clotting and growth factors, and kinins. Also active are the mediators released by Mast cells, Basophils and Platelets as well as the Eicosanoids generated by many cells at inflammatory sites, followed by Macrophages and Lymphocytes, wherever there is an immunological challenge.

The inflammatory process is very necessary and beneficial provided it is not too much or for too long. It is counter productive when it becomes chronic, causing unpleasant symptoms for the individual leading to excessive pain and swelling.

Aloe Vera's anti-inflammatory effects are as follows:

a) by the inactivation of Bradykinin due to a Carboxypeptidase enzyme, capable of hydrolising Bradykinin and Angiotensin 1 in vitro. Bradykinin acting at the site of acute inflammation is both a vasodilator and a potent pain producing agent. This may be the mechanism whereby pain is decreased by Aloe Vera, although this has not been properly demonstrated in vivo.

b) Aloe Vera contains Salicylic acid and also anthraquinones which can be broken down to form salicylates. Salicylates are both analgesic and anti-inflammatory, inhibiting the production of prostaglandins.

Delighted as I am with this result, I am aware that the problem recurs if I leave off the Aloe, for about a week, suggesting that it only suppresses the symptoms in this case, and is not a permanent cure for the problem.

My wife has noticed that after burning her hands on the AGA oven (her hobby is cooking), the swift application of Aloe Vera not only takes the pain away almost instantly, but with repeated applications the wounds heal much faster and without scarring. Previous burns have left her with multiple small scars on her hands and wrists but at least now she is not adding to them. Now you can see why it's called 'the Burn Plant'.

With experience my usage of Aloe Vera in my general medical practice has slowly increased over the two years, especially in areas where my usual treatment has failed or not been very successful, or where there have been side effects, or where the patient has asked for 'something natural'.

In practice the skin conditions I have found responded best are:

Acne vulgaris and rosacea
Eczema, especially (atopic) eczema in young children
Seborrhoeic dermatitis
Psoriasis
Chronic urticaria
Ulcers
Tinea pedis (athlete's foot)

An important observation that I personally made came about when I conducted a small experiment in treating a large ulcer on the shin of an elderly lady with just topical Aloe Vera; nothing else. This is probably just about the worst place to get an ulcer as traditionally, by whatever method is used, they can take a very long time to heal. I was excited to find an example that had just occurred as a result of trauma ~ she had knocked her leg against the sharp corner of some furniture. I saw it within a few hours of the accident happening and after cleaning the wound, persuaded my nursing staff to apply Aloe Vera twice a day under a moist dressing.

The speed of healing was quite remarkable with no sign of infection, which is the dreaded complication. I am pleased to say that the nurses were also impressed and would like to use it again on some of their cases which stubbornly refuse to heal. Quite remarkably this ulcer healed with minimal scarring, a typical feature of Aloe treatment.

If a result such as this is indeed consistent, then the Aloe Vera approach could save the National Health Service an awful lot of money.

Other workers also report excellent results with burns and ulcers and in the USA it is regularly used in some major burns units.

Wound Healing and Burns

Serious research into the wound healing qualities of Aloe Vera began in the 1930's after Collins and Collins reported in a 31 year old woman, a case of severe roentgen dermatitis with desquamation over an area 4 x 8cms of the forehead and extending above the hairline. Within 24 hours after the treatment with fresh Aloe the itching and burning had subsided completely. Within 5 weeks of continued treatment, there was complete regeneration of sensation and absence of a scar. After 3 months, there was no indication of a relapse and upon exposure to the sun, the forehead appeared to be pigmenting normally along with the other exposed skin surfaces.

Other experiments followed using both human and animal models where immediate and delayed histopathalogical changes of the skin in Aloe-treated and non Aloe-treated wounds could be observed. Many experiments were performed through the 1950's and 60's which consistently demonstrated further wound healing with greatly reduced scarring.

By the 1980's key workers like Professor John Heggars and Dr Wendel Winters in the USA working in academic plastic surgery units were putting forward hypotheses on the mechanisms of the anti-inflammatory and anti-thermal burn effects.

Their conclusions were that Aloe Vera was able to block the formation Thromboxane A2 which improved tissue survival following either burn or frostbite injury. This was brought about by a significantly increased dermal perfusion after the burn, given that Thromboxane A2 is a vasoconstrictor. Immunohistochemical assessment of the burnt material showed markedly decreased levels of

Thromboxane A2 in treated groups when compared with untreated controls. Robson et al in 1982 also showed Aloe Vera's ability to inhibit prostaglandin and thomboxane production. They noticed an absence of thromboxane B2 up to 72 hours post burn and a decrease in PGF2 levels up to the same time.

Thromboxanes and Prostaglandins are known to effect:

    i)   platelet aggregation
    ii)   leukocyte adherence
    iii)   vasoconstriction

In Japan since 1976, Professor Keisuke Fujita has been studying the Bradykininase activity in a natural Aloe - Aloe Vera Arborescens. He concluded that the anti-inflammatory enzyme he described was a serine carboxypeptidase which hydrolysed Bradykinin and Angiotensin I, a vasopressor, in vitro.

A later paper from 1993, reinforced the view that this enzyme is one of the key factors involved in the pharmacological effectiveness of Aloe. Aloe also contains Salicylic acid which is both analgesic and anti-inflammatory due to the inhibition of prostaglandin synthesis.

Other agents which also contribute to the anti-inflammatory effect, found by the Japanese workers, are thought to be plant hormones, Lectin like substances such as Aloctin A found by Saito et al in 1982.

One of the most satisfying aspects of general practice is that we get to know our patients and share with them some of the intimate and often amusing events in life. For example, I once gave an elderly gentleman some Aloe for this arthritis and asked to see him two weeks later. When he returned he looked happy and so I suggested that the Aloe must have improved his condition. "No," he said. "it's about the same - but I whistle when I walk now and my wife says that I haven't done that for twenty years."

Another chap, a retired dustman, stopped me in the street to tell me how pleased he was that I'd given his wife some Aloe to help her asthma. "It's improved it then, has it?" I asked, to which he replied "Yeah, her asthma is great, Doc', but so's my sex life - she can't get enough of me!"
"I'm really pleased for you," I said, trying hard not to smile as I noticed two litres of Aloe Vera gel in his shopping basket.

Aloe Vera is extremely safe and non-toxic and I think that virtually all people who react to Aloe Vera are probably reacting to the vehicle or additives necessary to preserve it. Of course, someone, somewhere must be allergic to Aloe Vera but, throughout the years, it has consistently been reported as very safe. Most commonly, allergic reactions are due to such added substances as lanolin or parabens in the creams, sandalwood or propolis itself. I have seen only one reaction to a drink, that was a hyperactive effect, the most likely culprit being the sodium benzoate used as a preservative.

The leading authority on toxicology in this country is the Poisons Unit at Guy's Hospital in London and, when asked about Aloe Vera, they admitted they had very little on file, only that some whole leaf products had been shown to produce abdominal pains and diarrhoea in some people. (I will explain the difference between the gel and whole leaf Aloe juice in a later chapter.)

I believe the only possible source of toxicity would be the anthraquinone fraction; in high concentration. But this level does not exist in the products sold as tonics or health drinks, and I believe them to be perfectly safe. Aloe Vera preparations have been sold in the USA for many years and, before going on sale to the general public, any American product has to pass the strict Food and Drugs Administration tests for safety before it can be sold as a food, in which group it is classed. No products are licensed yet to be sold as medicines in the UK.

Allergy to Aloe Vera

Only one form of pure reaction to Aloe Vera has been documented and that is discoid or Nummular Eczema following ingestion of the gel.

I have not discussed the use of Aloe Vera in cosmetics where it is designed to nourish the skin and retard the effects of ageing. It is widely used and the 'with Aloe Vera' handle is becoming much more common. Boots the Chemist and Body Shop have used it for a while, but recently Gillette has added Aloe Vera to one of their products to make shaving more pleasant for men. The combination of high quality Aloe in skin preparations firstly helps to moisturise and smooth the skin. It penetrates the skin, bringing about anti-inflammatory and anti-ageing effects, this includes the reduction and sometimes eradication of 'liver spots' on older skin.

Reduced Pigment Formation

Melanin is formed from the amino acid Tyrosine which is converted by the enzyme Tyrosinase to Dihydroxyphenylalanine (DOPA). This is then polymerised to form melanin. Aloe Vera through its anthraquinone fraction possesses anti-tyrosinase activity thereby reducing skin pigmentation. A preparation containing Aloesin is sold in the Far East for the sole purpose of lightening Asian skin.

Secondly, after penetration, it stimulates the fibroblasts in the dermis to produce more collagen and elastin, thereby reducing the tendency to wrinkles which occur as a result of reduced collagen levels. Finally, it enhances skin's immune system and therefore lessens the tendency to damage from ultraviolet rays.

Finally, before leaving the subject of skin it must be said that even Aloe Vera can have some side effects but, far from being harmful, they are generally welcomed. Women in particular, after several weeks of using the gel, often remark that their nails grow faster, and are not so brittle; that their hair also grows faster and looks healthier and that because Aloe Vera has a vasodilatory effect (opening the blood vessels in the skin) they can develop rosy cheeks. People who are told they look well, generally feel well.

The Digestive Tract

The other major organ system where Aloe consistently helps is in the digestive tract, from simple dyspepsia or indigestion and heartburn, to reported cases of it healing peptic ulcers, but I have no personal experience of the latter. Many ulcers are now known to be due to bacterium called Helicobacter Pylori and it would be interesting to see what effect Aloe Vera has on this bug. (I am trying to organise some in vitro testing at the time of writing.) If it were to be seen to kill this organism and bring about the healing of these ulcers, we would see an explosion in the demand for Aloe Vera and it would save the National Health Service the huge amount of money spent on courses of antibiotics used to eradicate the organism.

As I've said, in the past, Aloe Vera was used widely as a purgative and an aid to digestion generally, so it is not surprising that sufferers from inflammatory bowel conditions like colitis and diverticulitis have reported great results with regular ingestion of Aloe Vera. It must be stressed, however, that their symptoms tend to return after stopping the drink so taking Aloe Vera gel has to be an on-going habit. These conditions are well known for relapsing and remitting, and for some people who have suffered regularly from these unpleasant complaints, the reduced frequency and severity of the relapses has been benefit enough. I am often asked if Aloe Vera is available as a suppository but, as far as I'm aware, it is not as yet - but perhaps it's in the pipeline!!

One condition that I think deserves special mention is the irritable bowel syndrome (IBS). It is the commonest disorder of the bowel in the industrialised western world and the most frequent cause for referral to gastroenterologists by family doctors. It is estimated that there may be more than five million sufferers in the UK alone.

Irritable bowel syndrome is a collection of symptoms that vary from person to person but the most common features are abdominal pains, constipation or diarrhoea with abdominal bloating or with the passage of mucous. There is no effect on general health and the sufferers usually maintain their weight. But it can be an extremely debilitating and embarrassing condition, and can at times prevent sufferers from going outside and getting on with their work or, indeed, their life. Often it is associated with a stress-related emotional upset or depression and may be combined with other 'irritable' organs such as the bladder.

Conventional treatment is not terribly effective and depends on dietary change, usually with an increase in fibre, antidiarrhoeal or bulking agents, antispasmodic drugs, antidepressants and psycho/hypnotherapy, etc. All these measures are tried because the condition is not fully understood. Some think it is due to a disorder of the bowels' regular and smooth peristaltic movements - a 'dysmotility', and on the same theme others claim that the gut's sensitivity is decreased. Another theory is that there is too much yeast such as candida albicans in the bowel which may be the underlying cause, whilst there is a group of doctors who, as with post-viral fatigue syndrome (to be discussed later), think it is wholly psychological and the result of the stresses of modern living.

Whatever the cause, it was stated in the British Medical Journal in January 1995: "No uniformly successful treatment exists for the Irritable Bowel Syndrome". I know that there are a lot of dissatisfied patients out there, for when the journalist, Hazel Courtney, wrote an article on IBS in the Daily Mail in 1994, featuring amongst others, my views on Aloe Vera, it generated 10,000 letters asking for more information.

Aloe Vera has now become my first line approach in the treatment of confirmed IBS and I have more success with this regime than any other. Unfortunately, it is not successful in every case and I suspect the failures tend to occur more where the emotional response to stress is greatest, i.e. there is less of a physical component. But it is really reassuring and pleasing to hear patients say, as one did, "I can go shopping now with confidence - it's great". Previously she could only shop where she had an intimate knowledge of where all the toilets were to be found.

I must emphasise that I am talking about Aloe Vera gel, not the old 'bitter aloes' made from the sap. This would produce quite different results!

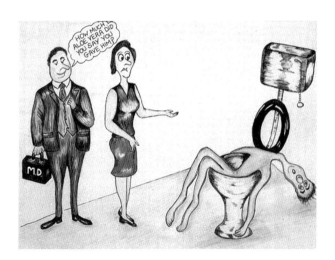

Immune system

People who take Aloe Vera gel regularly, including myself, report a greater sense of well-being - they just feel better and more at ease. I believe this comes about because of a well-balanced and effective immune system which the Aloe Vera is capable of modulating.

As the immune system exists to protect the body from change caused by invading organisms for example, bacteria, viruses or altered cells such as cancer cells, its efficient functioning is of extreme importance. It necessitates a very complex system, involving many different elements which I do not claim to fully understand. The study of immunology is a subject in its own right. So I will present it in a greatly over-simplified form, in which I shall mention only the key players. There is much more going on in the background which modifies the action of these key cells, as they do not work in isolation.

The immune system is working around the clock to protect the body from attack and therefore any disruption to its immediate and efficient response will cause a major problem to the individual. Problems can arise where the immune system is under active as well as when it is overactive, or even when there is inappropriate action such as when the system attacks the host tissues. This action will cause the so-called auto-immune disorders, some common examples being:

> Ulcerative colitis
> Systemic lupus erythematosus (lupus)
> Rheumatoid arthritis

If the immune system is unable to produce an adequate response, the individual can't fight infection and will eventually succumb. The classic instance of such a situation, of course, is AIDS or Acquired Immune Deficiency Syndrome.

If the response is too great, such as the hypersensitive response in allergic asthma, this is a harmful response capable of ultimately causing death, so it is vital that the response should be just enough to knock out the enemy without overkill.

Such immune responses are occurring in healthy individuals continuously. The immune system should be thought of as an essential part of our defence mechanism, continually keeping out and destroying invaders and abnormal cells as they appear.

Who are the key players?

The most important are cells called lymphocytes of which there are two types, B cells and T cells which are found in lymphoid tissue and in the blood.

Second in importance are cells called phagocytes which are basically scavengers. Some of these are found in tissue, while others which are the white blood cells, are found circulating in the blood. B lymphocytes produce antibodies but the T lymphocytes have several functions:

1. They help B cells to make antibodies
2. They recognise and destroy cells infected with viruses
3. They activate phagocytes to take up pathogens that they have identified
4. They control the level and quality of the immune response.

Life is a constant fight both internally and externally, so I have represented the immune response as a battle in which the orders are delivered by messengers. These messengers are called cytokines. The cytokine systems orchestrate the T helper cells (lymphocytes) in searching out and destroying the enemy and it is at this level where a major component of Aloe Vera works.

Lymphoid System

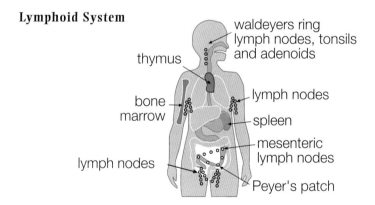

This very important component, acemannan, is found amongst the sugar fraction. It is a long chain polysaccharide and acts as an immune modulator. This means it has the ability to either enhance or to slow down the immune response and this remarkable activity has been demonstrated and is well documented in laboratory experiments.

It has been isolated from Aloe Vera by the Carrington Laboratories in the USA and produced as a drug, trade name 'Carrisyn', which has been licensed by the Food and Drugs Administration (FDA) to be trialled in human AIDS patients. Ace mannan has attracted enormous interest and the future of Aloe Vera may well be in the success of this component. At the moment it has reached the penultimate stage of testing before it can be licensed for unrestricted use in humans. It currently holds a veterinary licence in the USA for the treatment of feline leukaemia virus in cats.

On the veterinary side in the UK very recent work carried out by Peter Green, an equine vet, on post-viral syndrome in horses, has produced some dramatic results.

Fortunately, in equine post-viral syndrome, unlike that in human beings, there is a measurable entity in the blood. Horses with this condition drop their white blood cell counts to almost fatal levels. Peter Green recorded these levels in horses suffering from this condition, then put them on a three to five week regime of adding Aloe Vera gel to their feed. Being a sceptic at first - as I was - he was incredibly surprised with his findings as eleven out of fourteen horses treated made a full recovery and returned to eventing, jumping and racing. The affected horses all showed increased white cell counts after the course of Aloe Vera. Normally, most of these horses would not have expected to recover. In his paper Peter Green says: "Nevertheless, despite the limitations of this form of clinical study, we believe that there are genuine therapeutic benefits to be gained from the administration of Aloe Vera extracts".

I have suggested its use in my patients with post-viral fatigue syndrome on an empirical basis and one or two have benefited. However, the numbers are really too small to draw any conclusions but, considering there is no other convincing treatment, it must be worth a try.

On the basis of what has been said, it would be expected that those suffering with asthma of an allergic origin would benefit from Aloe Vera, either for the immunomodulating effect or the natural anti-inflammatory effect. In general, I have found this to be the case, leading to a reduction in the number of times they need to use their inhaler and the reduction in the frequency of severe disabling attacks. As with post viral syndrome I have not seen sufficient cases to be absolutely sure about it, but it certainly calls for some research - a topic I will return to at the end of the book.

Finally, on this subject, I must tell you Alison's story. The young woman to whom this book is dedicated and the patient who convinced me that there really was something worthwhile in Aloe Vera.

Alison is a delightful young woman whom I have treated for fifteen years. She suffers with Still's disease or juvenile rheumatoid arthritis. This condition has been progressive since she was a child and because of its severity and the deformity it has caused, she has been under regular specialist supervision and has received a variety of potent conventional treatments, both drug treatments including high-dose non-steroidal anti-inflammatory drugs (NSAIDS) and hydrotherapy. She has borne her disability bravely but about eighteen months ago she came to the surgery complaining that she needed more anti-inflammatories to control her pain and stiffness, but couldn't take any more because of the abdominal pain these caused. Catch 22. I didn't know what else to suggest so I said, "You wouldn't like to try a sort of wacky cactus juice that's supposed to have a natural anti-inflammatory effect as well as settling stomachs would you? Unfortunately, I can't prescribe it and you'll have to buy it from a local agent."

Alison and her mother, who was present during the consultation, said they would try anything to get some relief. So Alison started a course of Aloe Vera gel.

It was agreed that she would not reduce her current level of drugs but just add in the Aloe Vera and record the amounts of NSAIDS she took, the amount of Aloe Vera and her symptoms on a daily basis. I was to see her every two weeks.

After a few weeks we were both thrilled to see an improvement. Her abdominal pain disappeared, she was in less pain and she certainly looked better and happier - even to the extent of getting rosy cheeks for the first time. Over the subsequent months she started to reduce her NSAID level until, eighteen months down the road, she only takes about half the amount she used to, still with no side effects. Her quality of life has no doubt improved and witnessing this change, albeit in only one patient, but one of my most difficult therapeutically, was a turning point for me.

Thank you, Alison.

This kind of arthritis I suspect is helped by a combination of anti-inflammatory and immunomodulatory factors. However, Aloe Vera does seem to help the other 'wear and tear' type of arthritis - osteoarthritis, so the use of aloe in these cases must be worth investigating.

We have looked at acemannan but there are other aspects of polysaccharides, according to American nutritionist Dr E. Harendal, listed below. They are found in every single cell in the body and they play a crucial role by:

a)   lining the colon to prevent absorption of toxic waste
b)   providing a life-saving barrier against microbial invasion for each cell, especially viruses
c)   providing critical lubrication of joints
d)   helping to maintain the capacity of movement of fluids
e)   allowing the transfer of gases in the lungs
f)   facilitating the absorption of water, electrolytes and nutrients in the gastro Intestinal tract.

Dr Harendal believes they are as vital to a healthy body as bricks are to a house.

HOW DOES ALOE VERA WORK?

We know that an Aloe Vera leaf is approximately 99 per cent water. Therefore, the total amount of nutrient is in the remaining 1 per cent of the plant. In this 1 per cent, seventy-five ingredients form a cocktail of all the substances previously mentioned and in their relatively small amounts they would not be expected to have much effect, certainly not the results that have been witnessed. Why?

The answer I believe lies in their synergistic action. Synergism is defined as, "the working together of two or more drugs, muscles, etc., to produce an effect greater than the sum of their individual effects", and it is that balance that has taken thousands of years to evolve in this amazing plant and which produce its dramatic results.

Synergism in Phytotherapy

The scientific development of conventional or allopathic medicine required that the prescription drugs would be uniform chemical substances that would produce a consistent physiological effect. Hence the practice of isolating in chemically pure form the biologically active substances or "active ingredients" from botanical formulations. The tenet of the active ingredient is deeply ingrained in allopathic medicine.

Herbal preparations taken from whole stems, roots, leaves and fruits containing huge numbers of phytochemicals stretch the boundaries of the conventional medical paradigm.

The method of action is also often different whereas a cancer drug may kill cancer cells directly a herbal preparation may cause either the malignant cells to differentiate into normal, healthy cells or perhaps stimulate the body's immune system to better fight and destroy the abnormal cells.

Together with these views, Professor Henri Sharman, a physician from Ohio State University, believes that antioxidants work synergistically to neutralise free radicals, especially Vitamin C, Vitamin E, Carotene and various bioflavonoids. Ayruvedic herbal preparations are formulated just to maximise such synergistic action.

Complex herbal mixtures are more potent because they contain both water soluble and fat soluble antioxidants, therefore they are capable of scavenging free radicles both inside and outside the cell. It is also important to remember that natural-sourced and synthetic vitamins do not have the same composition nor the same biological activity. In respect of Vitamin E for example, studies have shown a preferential functional uptake and retention of the natural Vitamin E as compared to the synthetic form.

> Professor Sharman believes that herbal preparations have a synergistic multifaceted healing capacity, which warrants further systematic exploration for the benefit of humanity, leaving all preconceived notions behind.

This plant has the ability to:

(a) provide essential nutrients

Tissues that die and are renewed rapidly such as the lining of the gut, which renews itself about every four days, and the skin every twenty-one to twenty-eight days or so, need a rich and ready supply of building materials to produce and maintain healthy efficient cells. A poor diet and one which is deficient in certain key elements cannot produce a fit and healthy body (or mind come to that). It is becoming increasingly apparent that today's tendency to eat junk food, especially in children, is causing deficiency states that will produce a generation of unhealthy adults. An increasing number of doctors now emphasise that good nutrition is the basis of good health and that many diseases can be treated quickly and effectively by changes in diet rather than with drugs which generally only ameliorate the situation rather than effecting a cure.

Brillat Savarin (1755-1826), a Frenchman and gourmet, is always misquoted as saying, "You are what you eat". I tend to agree, but what he really said was, "Tell me what you eat, and I'll tell you who you are". This is more a social observation, but the truism lies in the misquotation. So it has been said that if the doctors of today don't become the nutritionists of tomorrow, then the nutritionists of today will become the doctors of tomorrow.

(b) kill bacteria, viruses, fungi and yeasts

In vitro experiments in the laboratory have been carried out on numerous organisms and have regularly shown that, in normal strength, Aloe Vera gel can kill or prevent replication of several bacterial organisms, such as:

Streptococcus pyogenes   Escherichia coli
Staphylococcus aureus   Propionibacterium acnes
Pseudamonas aeruginosa   Mycobacterium tuberculosis

The antimicrobial action of Aloe Vera was really first investigated in the USA between 1968-1972. Two doctors, Zimmerman and Sims, studied the effect of stabilised gel on:

Staphylococcus aureus   Streptococcus viridans
Candida albicans (yeast)   Corynebacterium xerosis

They found it inhibited growth of the bacteria at 70 per cent concentration and the yeast candida at a 50 per cent concentration.

Later, in 1970, they tested it against the fungi which cause athlete's foot (tinea pedis).

Trychophyton mentagrophytes is one such fungus. and another very stubborn fungus that can infect nails is Trychophyton rubrum. In concentrations of 85 per cent or more these fungi were killed. Further testing showed it to be virucidal against Herpes simplex and zoster (shingles).

In 1971, it was shown to kill Trichomonas vaginalis, a common cause of sexually transmitted vaginal infection producing soreness and discharge.

In her summary, Dr Sims reported, "Aloe Vera is bactericidal to at least six species of bacteria, especially to the more common staph and strep infections... It is timely in its use on burn patients. In an 80 per cent concentration, it is broadly virucidal. It is virucidal to four members of the Herpes strain, including Herpes simplex and Herpes zoster. In an 80 per cent concentration it is fungicidal against yeast infections, Trichomonas and Candida."

Aloe Vera gel has therefore the ability to kill organisms that particularly invade damaged skin and wounds, for if infection is present in the skin it will certainly delay healing, if not prevent it.

(c) reduce inflammation

Inflammation is the response of healthy tissues to injury. It is a complicated but organised process, involving changes in the local blood supply. The walls of the blood vessels change so that molecules and cells of the immune system may pass through them and then bring about clotting, mount an attack on pathogens and start repair.

If, however, the inflammatory response is too great, as for example in a hypersensitive reaction in allergic asthma, it will have an adverse effect and cause further tissue damage. If the inflammation is also inappropriate as when the body's own tissues are attacked, say in rheumatoid arthritis, it will aggravate the problem. This severe condition is generally treated with synthetic drugs to reduce inflammation and thereby pain and stiffness - the non-steroidal anti-inflammatory drugs, as used by Alison. A common N.S.A.I.D is the over the counter drug Ibuprofen. They are highly effective in reducing symptoms but, unfortunately, they often produce unacceptable side effects such as indigestion at one end of the scale, to bleeding stomach ulcers at the other.

A report that appeared in the British medical press in November 1995, suggested that some 5 per cent of duodenal, and a massive 22 per cent of gastric ulcers were associated with non-steroidal anti-inflammatory drugs, yet they are prescribed in their millions. So it should be a godsend to find a natural anti-inflammatory agent that works without the possibility of these horrific side-effects.

The combination of provision of nutrients, reduction in infection and inflammation, where appropriate, leads to promotion of new cell growth and more rapid healing. In a simple laboratory experiment in 1988, Danhof and McAnally added Aloe Vera gel to human fibroblast cell cultures. They saw an eight-fold increase in their replication, over control cultures to which no Aloe Vera had been added.

I have actually studied this paper in detail and it is apparent that their methods were flawed and I believe their results to be unreliable. Most other workers in this field looking at Aloe's effect on cell replication consistently find only a three to four fold increase, but this is remarkable enough.

Fibroblasts are one of the most important types of cells involved in the healing process. They produce the collagen fibres of the scar tissue that knit wounds together so the more that are working at the site of injury the better. This may be the single most important factor influenced by Aloe Vera in the acceleration of the healing process.

WHAT KIND OF ALOE?

The most fitting description is, I believe, was supplied by that American physician, Dr Ivan Danhof, who said, "The best Aloe is a preparation which maximises the desired constitutents, minimises any ingredient with negative effects, maintains the constituents in an unaltered and active form, preserves the actions and benefits, and is present in the final product in amounts which, indeed, can bring about the desired result when the product is used as recommended."

For the present I believe that the best form of Aloe is 100 per cent stabilised Aloe Vera gel as a health drink and that this stablised gel should be the major ingredient of any topical product such as shampoos, creams and ointments, lotions and sprays.

Aloe Vera is currently grown commercially mainly in the Rio Grande Valley in Texas, USA, in the Philippines, the Dominican Republic, South Africa, Spain and in Australia. There are several Aloe companies marketing a variety of Aloe compounds, some excellent and some I believe are absolutely useless. For any Aloe Vera drink to stand any chance of doing some good, I feel it must contain the parenchymatous gel and some sap. Therefore, it must possess a yellow or orange colour due to the sap, and taste bitter. If a product is clear, looks like water and tastes like water, then it probably is water!

There is a regulatory body based in the USA called the International Aloe Science Council and, amongst other things, it evaluates the quality of Aloe products. If such products, according to several criteria, reach a standard they are accredited with the IASC seal of approval, as below. This mark of quality can then appear on the container and I suggest that any Aloe product whose company does not display this seal of approval rather than just claiming to have it, has to be suspect.

I have listed below the various types of Aloe Vera products that may appear on the market, as defined by the IASC:

Raw Aloe Vera gel/juice - Naturally occurring unprocessed, undiluted parenchymatous tissue obtained from the decorticated (peeled) leaves of Aloe Barbadensis Miller (Aloe Vera Linne), and to which no other material has been added.

Aloe Vera gel/juice - Naturally occurring, processed undiluted, parenchymatous tissue obtained from the decorticated leaves of Aloe Barbadensis Miller, and to which no more than 5 per cent additives, including preservatives, shall be added as part of the processing.

Whole leaf Aloe Vera gel/juice - The whole leaf of the Aloe Barbadensis Miller including the rind and parenchymatous tissue that is processed, filtered and undiluted, to which no more than 5 percent additives, including preservatives shall be added as part of the processing.

Stabilized Aloe Vera gel/juice - Synonymous with the term Aloe Vera gel/juice. 100 per cent Aloe Vera (this definition for testing purposes only) - Processed, preserved liquid derived from the leaves of Aloe Barbadensis Miller (Aloe Vera Linne), and defined by a value using the reporting procedure adopted by the IASC.

Aloe Vera gel/juice spray dried - Aloe Vera gel/juice that has been spray dried with or without a matrix.

Reconstituted Aloe Vera gel/juice spray dried - Aloe Vera gel/juice spray dried to which an appropriate amount of water is added to achieve a concentration that is equivalent to 100 per cent Aloe Vera as defined.

Aloe Vera gel/juice freeze dried - Aloe Vera gel/juice that has been freeze dried with or without a matrix.

Reconstituted Aloe Vera gel/juice freeze dried - Aloe Vera gel/juice freeze dried to which an appropriate amount of water is added to achieve a concentration that is equivalent to 100 per cent Aloe Vera gel/juice as defined.

Aloe Vera concentrate - Aloe Vera gel/juice from which natural water has been mechanically removed to a desired level.

Reconstituted Aloe Vera gel/juice - Aloe Vera concentrate to which an appropriate amount of water is added to achieve a concentration that is equivalent to 100 per cent Aloe Vera as defined.

Aloe Vera beverage - An ingestible product containing a minimum of 50 per cent Aloe Vera juice as defined by the reporting procedure adopted by the IASC.

Aloe Vera drink - An ingestible product containing more than 10 per cent of Aloe Vera juice as defined by the reporting procedure adopted by the IASC.

Aloe Vera pulp - The parenchymal tissue and fibre derived from raw Aloe Vera gel/juice.

Aloe Vera oil - The lipid (fatty) portion obtained from the rind of the leaves of Aloe Barbadensis Miller by various solvent extract processes.

Aloe USP - The dried latex of the leaves of Aloe Barbadensis Miller (Aloe Vera Linne), known in commerce as Curacao Aloe or Aloe Ferox Miller and hybrids of this species with Aloe Africana Miller and Aloe Spicata Baker known in commerce as Cape Aloe (Lilaceae).

Aloe Vera latex - The bitter yellow liquid contained in the pericyclic tubules of the rind of Aloe Barbadensis Miller including the rind and internal portions of the plant.

Cold stabilised Aloe Vera gel, which is my preferred preparation, is about 97 per cent pure and the nearest thing that one can get to the natural raw gel extracted from the plant. As I have said, it is extremely safe and non-toxic, although when people first start to take the gel it often stirs them up and they may experience a change in bowel habit for a few days, together with slight abdominal discomfort, but this generally soon passes. Some people refer to this initial phase as one of detoxification but I think this is a misnomer. There is also a method of heat stabilisation, or pasteurisation, but this destroys some of the nutrients and enzymes so I believe we must aim to find the nearest thing to the natural, raw gel.

Please note that a product containing only 15 per cent Aloe Vera gel by volume can legally be called 100 per cent Aloe Vera juice.

Currently, the main debate centres on the relative benefits of Aloe Vera gel versus whole leaf Aloe.

In the production of whole leaf Aloe products, the whole plant is harvested, rather than individual leaves, and it is crushed. Solid matter, including the pulverised rind is separated and the resultant fluid is filtered through carbon filters to remove the excess anthraquinones and, in some cases, all of them. It is often then concentrated because a smaller number of plants is required for a given amount of product and there is less weight, due to its concentration, so reducing transport costs. The final product is cheaper at retail. It is often suggested that it is better because it contains more polysaccharides (coming from the inner rind) than the gel/sap only products, but I believe there are flaws in this argument and I would ask the following questions:

Polysaccharides are sugars that have formed a bond with water. What happens to them when water is removed during the concentration process? Do they possess the same biochemical qualities when reconstituted? Some manufacturers argue that by including the amount of polysaccharides in their products they must therefore be more powerful. I do not believe this is to be so because the digestive tract, due to the special way that polysaccharides are absorbed through the pinocytosis, can only handle so much, Once absorbed the body can also only utilise so much. The optimum concentration for absorption is that found in the natural gel at circa 1000 - 1200 mg/litre.

When the fluid is passed through the fine carbon filters during the manufacturing process, could unknown and unidentified important elements be filtered out as well?

As there is no real evidence for the time being, to support whole leaf Aloe being superior to 100 per cent stabilised Aloe Vera gel, I will go for this one. I believe that many of the considerations that go into making the whole leaf Aloe are really commercial, to get a cheaper product with a greater profit margin into the market place, The choice is yours.

The case for Aloin (Barbaloin) and against filtration

Activated carbon will attract and hold any molecules that have an electrical charge created by a double bond of the carbon in the molecule to other atoms. Molecules with an outside double bond are strongly "adsorbed" by carbon filters which means that Aloin and Aloe-emodin both containing such bonds are effectively trapped and removed by them. However, a large number of beneficial components in Aloe also contain outside double bonds and will be therefore filtered out. Among these are the glycoproteins (enzymes), proteins, mineral salts, all essential amino acids, Vitamins B1, B2, B6, B12, folic acid, carotene, various fatty acids and salicylic acid. Carbon filters also have an affinity for carbon itself therefore they may attract organic molecules regardless of their polarity. Polysaccharides are not removed by carbon filtration but many important elements are either completely taken out or their amounts are considerably reduced.

Why have aloin in a product anyway? When it has been suggested that it may be carcinogenic and produce abortions when taken orally, or kill fibroblasts when applied topically.

As with many substances, Parcelsus (1500 AD) knew that "the poison is in the dose". Whereas large amounts of aloin or other anthraquinones especially those with an amino or nitro group in them may prove harmful over a prolonged period of time; although there is no real evidence to support this, I believe that in small quantities aloin is actually a beneficial component of Aloe drinks. Aloin by the way, possesses hydroxyl groups, rather than the suspect nitro or amino groups.

Many, if not most workers in the field now believe that a small amount of aloin <50 ppm in a product improves the absorption of the other Aloe elements as well as being an important anti-microbial agent enabling Aloe to regulate the gut flora. Aloin is broken down eventually to form salicylates which are anti-inflammatory. It may also act as a trigger to the polysaccharides, working synergistically with them to enhance their various effects.

In topical products aloin and the other anthraquinone derivatives are anti-microbial, anti-inflammatory and also have anti-tyrosinase action, blocking melanin formation. They can also block ultraviolet light when applied topically.

ALOE IN THE FUTURE

Since earliest time, Aloe Vera has occupied a prominent place in medicinal folklore of various cultures. In small doses it was used as a general tonic and in large doses as a purgative. It was also used to treat indigestion, to get rid of intestinal parasites and worms. It was favoured as an insecticide and as an antiseptic and, most importantly, as a way of healing ulcerated, burnt, infected, lacerated and generally damaged skin whether from internal or external causes.

The use of Aloe Vera as a beauty aid is rapidly increasing. But why is it not being prescribed more by doctors? Perhaps they are not aware of it, and if that is the case I hope this book will go some way to promoting thought and further enquiry amongst my colleagues.

The main reason has to be the lack of hard evidence, i.e., evidence that is accepted by the body of the profession, be they GPs or specialists - the randomised double-blind clinical trial. This kind of clinical trial is the definitive way of assessing whether a new treatment actually works and is superior to other treatments. It involves the selected patients to be divided into two groups. One group receives only a placebo or another form of treatment and the other group receives the treatment under test. It is essential that neither the patient nor the doctor knows which treatment is being prescribed so there can be no bias. Only when the trial is completed are the different treatments revealed and the results analysed.

Until recently the documented trials were, regrettably, not of the quality and precision that would win over the sceptical, scientifically orientated doctor, especially with the current emphasis of evidence based medicine. The overwhelming anecdotal evidence has largely been ignored by regular practitioners, but fortunately there are some who have given it a try. I know of a handful of doctors, both in the National Health Service and private sector who now regularly use Aloe in their practices.

One small but significant trial was carried out in 1985, by Dr Jeffrey Bland, a nutritionist of the Linus Pauling Institute of Science and Medicine in California. He studied the effect of Aloe Vera on the gastrointestinal function in normal humans and involved ten volunteers, five of each sex. They changed nothing in their lifestyle but consumed two ounces of Aloe Vera juice three times a day for seven consecutive days.

Before entering the study the participants fasted overnight so that base line gastric secretion could be measured by a pH (level of acidity) sensitive capsule. After their gastric pH was measured, morning stool and urine samples were collected. The object of the experiment was to see if Aloe had any effects on these two functions. Dr Bland looked at urinary indican, which reflects the bowel bacterial conversion of the amino acid tryptophan and therefore possible improved protein digestion and absorption after Aloe Vera treatment. He also looked at stool specific gravity, gastric pH and bowel motility.

He found that urinary indican levels after one week on Aloe were lowered, suggesting an increase in both protein breakdown and absorption. He also found stool specific gravity was reduced with a faster movement of stool through the bowel, both suggesting an increase in water in the stool. No diarrhoea was reported. He also found the pH was normalised or buffered, meaning that Aloe Vera acted as an alkalising agent.

He commented that the Aloe Vera had helped to normalise stool bacterial cultures in six subjects, four of the six having previously had high yeast levels in their gut.

In discussing his findings, Jeffrey Bland said:

"The tolerance of the subjects to Aloe Vera juice supplementation was in general quite good. One person complained of gas and another of transient gut pain which after continued supplementation throughout the week, diminished. The other eight subjects were asymptomatic with no diarrhoea, nausea, intestinal bloating or distress. Four of the subjects noted an improved bowel regularity with greater gastrointestinal comfort after eating. Three indicated that they felt some enhancement of energy and a sense of well-being, although this could not be confirmed quantitatively."

It must be noted because the Food and Drugs Administration regard Aloe Vera as a food, the gel in the USA must be referred to as juice.

Although the scale of this experiment is too small to be of real significance, I believe it does highlight, in a semi-controlled fashion, the experiences that are repeatedly talked of anecdotally and it reinforces the need for further investigation on a larger scale.

The most important trials to appear recently were published by T Syed et al; one on Psoriasis in the Journal of Tropical Medicine and International Health and the other on Genital herpes in the Journal of Dermatological treatment.

Both fitted the necessary criteria being randomised double blind and controlled and showed impressive results. They achieved an 83% cure rate with Aloe in Psoriasis against a 6% rate with the control. In the Herpes trial there was 66.7% healing as opposed to 6.7% with the control. To establish the validity beyond doubt these results must be repeated by other workers in other clinical trials elsewhere.

Professor Edzard Ernst, Director of the Centre for Complementary Health Studies at Exeter University with whom I have had discussions also feels Aloe should be formally investigated. But, regrettably, clinical trials are expensive and they require willing consultants to undertake them. If a pharmaceutical company thought there was money to be made out of Aloe, then funding would be forthcoming, but for them it would be pointless as they could never achieve a patent!

However, I believe the future of Aloe Vera is rosy because there is a definite move in the community towards natural remedies and the medical profession is beginning to recognise this and slowly adapt.

Complementary medicine is undeniably a major growth area. In the UK 15 per cent of non-hospital consultations are now with complementary therapists whose numbers have mushroomed from 2,900 in 1981, to more than 60,000 at the last count. But the UK still lags behind most European countries and the United States, where visits to complementary therapists exceed those to conventional doctors.

Recently published in the British Medical Journal, the official organ of the British Medical Association, in a series of articles on this change towards complementary and over the counter medicines were some most interesting statistics.

Market breakdown for major categories of non-prescription medicines:

Pain	£196.4m	(1 6.7%)
Skin	£143.5m	(1 1.3%)
Cold	£93.9m	(7.4%)
Cough	£68.1m	(5.4%)
Sore throat	£72.7m	(5.7%)
Indigestion	£73.9m	(5.8%)
Total	£1268.5m	

Everyday ailments for which people report treating themselves rather than seeking a consultation with a doctor:

Ailment	Percentage of people reporting ailment (n=2000)
Headache	80
Athlete's foot	79
Dandruff	73
Heartburn	62
Migraine	62
Period pain	61
Colds	60
Coughs	56
Mouth ulcers	51
Acid stomach	50

The article concluded with a comment that has two implications for doctors.

If the scope of self medication widens as predicted, doctors, pharmacists, and other health professionals will need to respond in a more active and constructive way than they have to date.
(BMJ Vol.312, 30/3/1996)

I am encouraged by interest shown in university departments at Oxford, both on the dermatology and gastroenterology departments, and there is a reasonable chance that proper trials looking at venous leg ulcers and IBS may be conducted there in the near future; watch out for the next edition!

Aloe Vera's eponym 'the Medicine Plant' is a fitting one and we must constantly remind ourselves of the influence that folklore has had on medicine over the ages and the plants that have provided powerful drugs once isolated - opium from the poppy, digitalis from the foxglove, ergot from rye, and aspirin from willow bark to name but a few.

"Within the infant rind of this weak
flower poison hath residence and medicine power."

Romeo and Juliet.

In fact, 121 prescription drugs in common use owe their origins to plants, being concocted from 95 separate plants.

Eighty-eight per cent of people in developing countries rely on plant extracts for primary health care. In Africa where the AIDS pandemic is most aggressive and from where Aloe Vera originated, GIFTS OF HEALTH (Global Initiative for Traditional Systems of Health), a charitable organisation, is considering a project to develop Aloe and educate the people to use it, amongst other things to treat genital herpes. It has been shown to be effective against this virus whose lesions often form the portal of entry of the HIV virus and so by reducing the effects of genital herpes one can similarly reduce the incidence of AIDS.

Most plant species are to be found in rainforests of which 400,000 hectares, or the area of Scotland, are disappearing every week so by 2000 AD, 10 per cent of the world's 250,000 species of plant could be extinct.

I will leave you to ponder on this and suggest the following two quotations:

"The Doctor of the future will give no medicine but
will interest his patients in the care of the human frame, in diet
and in the cause and prevention of disease".

Thomas A Edison
1847 - 1931
American Inventor

" ...and above all do no harm."

Hippocrates

FURTHER READING

1   **Aloe Vera**
Carole Miller Kent. Arlington, Virginia
The Print Factory, 1979

2   **Aloe Vera Heals - The Scientific Facts**
K. Gottlieb. Denver, Colorado.
Royal Publications Inc., 1980

3   **The Silent Healer**
Bill Coats. 1984

4   **Remarkable Aloe - Aloe through the Ages**
Ivan E. Danhof PhD. M.D.
Omnimedicus Press, 1987

5   **Aloe - Myth Magic Medicine**
Odus M. Hennessee
Universal Graphics. Lawston O.K. 73502 1990

6   **Aloe Vera The Natural Healer**
Paul Hornsey-Pennell
Wordsmith Publishing Company, 1994

7   **Aloe Vera - The Inside Story**
Bill Coats 1995.

8   **Aloe Vera - The Health and Healing Plant**
Ed. Maykut and Marc Schweitzer, 1995

GLOSSARY

Acne
Skin disease characterised by pustules and cysts especially on the face.

Vulgaris   - occurring in adolescents and young adults.
Rosacea   - occurring in middle age and producing redness of nose and cheeks.

Amino Acids
Group of organic nitrogen containing compounds that form the component molecules of proteins.

Anthraquinones
A complex of phenolic substances which can be found in the sap of Aloe Vera acknowledged to have both pain killing, antibacterial and viruscidal activity. They also exhibit powerful laxative effects in their pure form.

Bioflavonoid
Any of a group of biologically active substances found widely in plants. Also called 'Vitamin P'.

Antioxidant
A group of substances including certain Vitamins, Minerals and Micronutrients which counter the activity of free radicals, inhibiting their ability to oxidise.

Catalyst
A substance that increases the rate of a chemical reaction without itself suffering any permanent chemical change.

Carbohydrates
A large group of organic compounds including sugars and starch that contain carbon, hydrogen and oxygen. They are a source of food and energy for animals.

Candida Albicans
A yeast like parasite fungus that causes the condition known as 'thrush'.

Colitis
An inflammatory condition of the colon or large bowel.

Collagen
A fibrous protein occurring in bone, cartilage and connective tissue.

Crohn's Disease
An inflammatory disease of the small bowel otherwise called regional ileitis.

Dalton
A unit of measurement named after the British chemist John Dalton (1766-1844).

Dermabrasion
Method of treating scarred skin by surgically removing the damaged epidermis.

Diverticulosis
A condition in which diverticulae in the colon are associated with lower abdominal pain.

Dysmotility
Disorder of movement, causing irregular spasms of the bowel leading to abdominal pain.

Eczema
A non-contagious inflammation of the skin, marked usually by redness, itching and weeping lesions which become encrusted and scaly. Usually found in dry skin.

Elastin
A protein that is the principal component of elastic tissue found in the walls of arteries, the dermis of the skin and other elastic structures.

Enzyme
Any of the numerous proteins produced by living organisms and functioning as biochemical catalysts.

Epithelium
A layer of cells that covers the body or lines a cavity that connects with it.

Fibroblast
A cell in connective tissue that is responsible for producing fibres and is most important in the healing process.

Free Radical
An atom or group of atoms containing at least one unpaired electron, existing for a brief period of time before reacting to produce a stable molecule.

Immune System
A series of cells found in the blood, tissues and lymphoid system which protects the body from attack by micro-organisms and altered cells such as cancer cells.

Irritable Bowel Syndrome
A functional bowel disorder in which abdominal pain is associated with defaecation or change in bowel habit or abdominal distension.

Lignin
A complex polymer of cellulose occurring in certain plant cell walls making the plant rigid. When applied to the skin in a topical cream it bestows an ability to penetrate, carrying accompanying elements with it.

Lymphocyte
A white blood cell, part of the immune system, found in the blood and lymphoid tissue.

Metabolism
The sum of the chemical processes that occur in living organisms resulting in growth, production of energy and elimination of waste, etc.

NSAID
A group of drugs used in the treatment of arthritis, achieving their effect by the inhibition of prostaglandin synthesis. All can cause gastrointestinal irritation.

Phagocyte
Cells found in the blood and tissue which can engulf and digest other cells, microgranisms and other foreign bodies.

Pinocytosis
A process whereby microscopic particles are engulfed whole by cells

Placebo
A substance containing no active drug given to a patient usually to compare its effects with those of a real drug.

Polysaccharides
Long chain sugars that form chemical bonds with water to produce mucilaginous and lubricating fluids.

Propolis
A resinous aromatic substance collected by bees from the bark and buds of trees, used to line their hives thereby creating a sterile environment.

Protein
Organic compounds of high molecular weight that contain amino acids as their basic structural units. They are essential for the growth and repair of animal tissue.

Prostaglandin
A group of hormone like substances capable of stimulating the smooth muscle of the uterus or that in blood vessels.

Psoriasis
A chronic non-contagious skin disease characterised by inflammation and red, scaly patches. It can also cause a type of arthritis.

Saponins
Soapy substances, chemically glycosides which provide cleansing and antiseptic properties.

Seborrhoea
A disease of the skin characterised by excessive secretion of greasy material (sebum) leading to the formation of oily scales on the skin.

Synergism
The action of two or more substances to achieve an effect greater than the sum of their individual effects.

Systemic Lupus Erythematous (S.L.E. or Lupus)
A chronic inflammatory disease affecting the skin and internal organs.

Tinea Pedis
A fungal disease of the skin of the foot.

Urticaria
An acute or chronic disease of the skin causing intense itchiness associated with red, raised patches often associated with an allergic reaction to internal or external agents. Often referred to as 'Hives' or 'Nettlerash'.

PART II

RESEARCH BIBLIOGRAPHY

The research bibliography has been divided into sections for convenient use. In each section, the papers and articles are in alphabetical order by author and in chronological order where an author has written more than one paper. Where I consider work to be important, it appears in bold type. The importance attached to any work may reflect the subject matter, the calibre of the author or Institution or may just be of historical interest.

The vast majority of research into Aloe Vera tends to emphasise the positive attributes of the plant but there are, as one would expect, some negative ones.

Unfortunately, various similar studies involving Aloe preparations do not always produce consistent results. This outcome can probably be attributed to variability in the source of the Aloe plants, variability in the production process, or the presence in the preparations of multiple components with varying and even opposing biological activities. There is also the tendency to use different vehicles for delivering the aloe.

Most research carried out to date involves laboratory experiments or experiments with animals. Only a small proportion, describes human clinical trials but this pattern is changing as shown by some of the more recent work which which looks at Psoriasis, Diabetes Mellitus and Genital Herpes.

Very shortly, I hope to be able to add to the clinical trials when I publish work on Aloe Vera in the treatment of chronic various leg ulcers and in the Irritable Bowel Syndrome.

A short introduction to each section will point out areas of interest, concern or criticism so that the reader may quickly locate the required information from the considerable amount of material available.

SECTION I - EFFECT ON CELL GROWTH

The effect of Aloe Vera on cells is studied in two areas. (a) What is its effect on the growth of normal cells and (b) What is its effect on the growth of preneoplastic or frankly malignant cells.

When assessing this effect it is most important to look at which fraction of Aloe Vera is being tested. Is it the gel or is it largely the sap or phenolic (anthraquinone) fraction? Their effects are very different; in fact, they produce an opposite result.

Exposure to the gel stimulates the replication of normal cells, whereas the anthraquinones and their derivatives will retard cell growth or may kill them. Both fibroblasts and neuron-like cells have been tested and it has been shown that there is a significant increase in proliferation in vitro under the influence of gel extracts.

Hydroxyanthraquinones, those found in Aloe Vera, have not been found to be carcinogenic, but there is a question mark over some of the other members of this chemical group, e.g. where amino or nitro groups are involved. These have been shown to produce renal tumours in experimental rats though the effect on humans is still inconclusive. The break-down product in humans, Emodin, a phenolic anthraquinone, shows limited evidence of toxicity / carcinogenicity in experimental animals. This which is important when considering people who abuse laxatives such as Senna or Cascara in which the substances are found.

Bouthet, C.F.; Schirf, V.R.; Winters, W.D. Stimulation of neuron-like cell growth of Aloe substances. Phytother. Res. 1995. 9. 185-188.

Brasher, W.J.; Zimmermann, E.R.; Collings, C.K. The effects of Prednisolone, Indomethacin and Aloe Vera Gel on tissue culture cells, oral surgery, oral medicine and oral pathology. 1969. 27. 122-128.

Danhof I.E.; McAnalley, B.H. Stabilised Aloe Vera - effect on human skin cells Drug & Cosmetic Industry. 1983. 133. 52,54,105-106.

Jeong, H.Y.; Kim, J.H.; Hwang, S.J.; Rhee, D.K. Anticancer effects of Aloe on sarcoma 180 in ICR mouse and on human cancer cell lines. Yakhak Hoeji. 1994. 38(3). 311-321.

Nakasugi; Tohru; Komai; Koichiro. Antimutagen of Aloe plants (Anthraquinones - Aloe Emodin) Kinki Daigaku, Nogakubu, Kiyo. 1994. 27. 47-54.

Sendelbach, L.E. A Review of the Toxitcity and Carcinogenicity of Anthraquinone derivatives. Toxicology 1989. 57.227-240.

Tsuda, H.; Ito, M.; Hirono, I.; Kawai, K.; Beppu, H.; Fujita, K.; Nagao, M. Inhibitory effect of Aloe arborescens Miller var natalensis Berger on induction of preneoplastic focal lesions in the rat liver. International Congress of Phytotherapy. 1991, Oct. Seoul, Korea 53.

Tsuda, H.; Matsumoto, K.; Ibo, M.; Hiroto, I.; Kawai, K.; Beppu, H.; Fujita, K.; Nagao, M. Inhibitory effect of Aloe arborescens. Miller var. natalensis Berger (Kidachi Aloe) on induction of preneoplastic focal lesions in the rat liver. Phytotherapy Research. 1993. 7. (No Special Issue) 543-547.

Westendorf; Marquardt; Poginsky; Dominiak; Schmidt. Genotoxicity of naturally occurring Hydroxyanthraquinones. Evaluation of mutagenicity and cell-transforming activity. Mutat. Res. 1990 Jan. 240(1). 1-12.

Wimbus, W.D.; Benavides, R.; Clause, W.J Effects of Aloe extracts on human and tumour cells in-vitro. Econ. Bot. 1981. 35(1) 89-95.

Winters, W.D.; Benavides, R.; Clouse, W.J. Effects of Aloe Extracts on Human Normal and Tumor Cells In Vitro. Econ. Bot. 1981. 35: 89-95.

Wolfe, D.; Schmutgte, C.; Westendorf, J.; Marquardt, H. Hydroxyanthraquinones as tumour promoters: enhancement of malignant transformation of C3H mouse fibroblasts and growth stimulation of primary rat hepatocytes. Cancer Res. (USA). 1990 Oct. 50(20). 6540-6544.

SECTION II - ANTI-INFLAMMATORY EFFECT

Experimental work in this field has largely been carried about by the podiatrists (chiropodists) and one worker stands out above all others. He is Professor R.H. Davis, Professor of Physiology at the Pennsylvanian College of Podiatric Medicine. He has repeatedly demonstrated Aloe's anti-inflammatory effect, both on soft tissues and in arthritis. His work, however, is limited to animal experiments but he has not carried out any Clinical Studies on patients.

Afzal, M.; Ali, M.; Hassam, R.A.N.; Sweedan, N.; Dhami, M.S.I. Identification of some prostanoids in Aloe Vera extracts. Planta Medica. 1991. 57(1). 38-40.

Bradshaw, T.W. Aloe Vera: its influence on the physiology of wound healing and inflammation. J. Brit. Pod. Med. 1996. 51(2). 25-29. A7

Brasher, W.J.; Zimmermann, E.R.; Collings, C.K. The effects of Prednisolone, Indomethacin and Aloe Vera Gel on tissue culture cells, oral surgery, oral medicine and oral pathology. 1969. 27. 122-128.

Capasso, F.; Mascolo N.; Autore, G.; Duraccio, M.R. Effect of Indomethacin on Aloin and 1,8 Dioxianthraquinone-induced Production of Prostaglandins in Rat Isolated Colon. Prostglandins. 1983. 26. 557-562.

Davis R.H.; Didonato J.J.; Hartman G.M.; Haas R.C. Anti-Inflammatory and wound healing activity of a growth substance in Aloe Vera.J. Am. Podiatric Med. Assoc.1984 Feb. 84:.

Davis, R.H.; Agnew, P.S.; Shapiro, E. Antiarthritic activity of anthraquinones found in Aloe for podiatric medicine. J. Am. Podiatric Med. Assoc. 1986. 76(2) 61-66.

Davis, R.H.; Kabbani, J.M.; Maro, N.P. Aloe Vera and inflammations. Proc. Pa. Acad. Sci. 1986. (recd. 1987) 60(1) 67-70.

Davis, R.H.; Leitner, M.E.; Russo, J.M. Topical anti-inflammatory activity of Aloe Vera as measured by ear swelling. J. Am. Podiatric. Med. Assoc. 1987. 77(11) 610-612.

Davis, R.H.; Leitner, M.G.; Russo, J M; Byrne, M.E. Anti inflammatory activity of Aloe Vera against a spectrum of irritants. (Oral activity found to be dependent on presence of Anthraquinones). J. Am. Podiatric Med. Assoc. (US). 1989 June. 79 (6). 263-276.

Davis, R.H.; Maro, N.P. Aloe Vera and gibberellin. Anti-inflammatory activity in diabetes. J. Am. Podiatric Med. Assoc. 1989 Jan. 79 (1). 24-26.

Davis, R.H.; Rosenthal, K.Y.; Cesario, L.R.; Omu, G.A. Processed Aloe Vera administered topically inhibits inflammation. J. Am. Podiatric Med. Assoc. 1989. 79(8). 395-397.

Davis, R.H.; Parker, W.L.; Murdoch, D.P. Aloe Vera as a biologically active vehicle for hydrocortisone acetate. J.Am. Podiatric Med. Assoc.1991. 81(1). 1-9. A3

Davis, R.H. Influence of Aloe on inflammation and wound healing. International Congress of Phytotherapy. 1991 Oct. Seoul, Korea. 29.

Davis, R.H.; Stewart, G.J.; Bregman, P.J. Aloe Vera and the inflamed synovial pouch model. J. Am. Podiatric Med. Assoc. 1992 Mar. 82 (3). 140-148.

Davis, R.H.; Didonato, J.J.; Hartman, G.M.; Haas, R.C. Anti-inflammatory and wound healing activity of a growth substance in Aloe Vera. J. Am. Podiatric. Med. Assoc. 1994 Feb. 84(2). 77-81.

Davis, R.H.; Didonato, J.J.; Johnson, R.W.; Stewart, C.B. Aloe Vera, hydrocortisone and sterol influence on wound tensile strength and anti-inflammation. J. Am. Podiatric Med. Assoc. 1994 Dec. 84(12). 614-621.

Fujita, K.; Teradoura, R.; Nagatsu, T. Bradykinase activity of Aloe extract. Biochemical Pharmacology. 1976. 25. 205.

Fujita, K.; Ito, S.; Teradaira, R.; Beppu, H. Properties of carboxypeptidase from Aloe. Biochemical Pharmacology. 1979. 28. 1261-1262.

Ibo, S; Teradaira, R.; Beppu, H; Obata, M.; Nagatsu, T.; Fujita, K. Properties and pharmacological activity of carboxypeptidase in Aloe arborescens Miller var. natalensis Berger. International Congress of Phytotherapy. 1991 Oct. Seoul, Korea. 39.

Ibo, S; Teradaira, R; Beppu, H; Obata. M.; Fijita, K; Nagabsu, T. Biochemical properties of carboxypeptidase from Aloe arborescens Miller var. natalensis Berger. Phytotherapy Research. 1993. 7. No special issue. S26-29.

Ibo, S.; Teradaira, R.; Beppu, H.; Obata, M.; Fujita, K.; Nagatsu, T. Biochemical properties of Carboxypeptidase from Aloe arborescens Miller var. natalensis Berger. Phytother. Res. 1993. 7. S26-29. A2

Knight, J.H.; Stevens, E. Anti-inflammatory and healing properties of Aloe barbadensis. International Congress of Phytotherapy 1991 Oct. Seoul, Korea. 31.

Nakagomi, K.; Oka, S.; Tomizuka, N.; Yamamoto, N.; Masui, T.; Nakazawa, H. A novel biological activity in Aloe components effects on mast cell degranulation and platelet aggregation. Rep. Ferment Res. Inst. (Yakabie) 1985. 0(63). 23-30.

Obata, M.; Ibo, S.; Beppu, H.; Fujita, K.; Nagatou, T. Mechanism of anti-inflammatory and antithermal burn action of CPase from Aloe arborescens Miller var natalensis Berger in rats and mice. Phytother. Res. 1993. 7. Special issue. 530-533.

Udupa, S.L.; Udupa, A.L.; Kulkarmi, D.R. Anti-inflammatory and wound healing properties of Aloe Vera. Fitoterapia. 1994. 65(2). 141-145.

Vamamoto, M.; Sugyama, K.; Voketa, M.; Maeda, Y.; Nakagomi, K.; Nakazawa, H. Inhibitory effects of Aloe extracts on antigen and compound 48-80 induced histamine release from rat peritoneal mast cells. Japanese Journal of Toxicology and Environmental Health. 1993. 39(5). 395-400.

Yagi, A.; Harada, N.; Yamada, H.; Iwadare, S.; Nishioka, I. Antibradykinin active material in Aloe saponaria. Journal of Pharmaceutical Science. 1982 b. 71. 1172-1174.

Yamamoto, M;. Sugiyama, K.; Yokota, M.; Maeda, Y.; Nakagomi, K.; Nakazawa, H. Inhibitory effects of Aloe extracts on antigen and compound 48-80 induced histamine release from rat peritoneal mast cells. Japanese Journal of Toxicology and Environmental Health. 1993. 39(5) 395-400.

SECTION III - ANTI-MICROBIAL EFFECT

Extracts of Aloe Vera have been shown to possess anti-bacterial, anti-viral and anti-fungal/yeast effects. This action is mediated by both the gel and the sap but by far the most potent in vitro effects are seen by the anthraquinones in the sap. Whereas in vitro the anti-viral effects are mediated through the long chain sugars which can be consumed orally or injected.

Andersen, D.C.; Weber, N.D.; Wood, S.G.; Hughes, B.G.; Murray, B.K.; North, J.A. In vitro virucidal activity of selected anthraquinones and anthraquinone derivatives. Antiviral. Res. 1991. Sep. 16(2). 185-96.

Benigni, R.; Substances with antibiotic action contained in anthraquinonic drugs. Chem. Ab. 1950. 44. 11036.

Bruce, W.G.G. Investigations of the anti-bacterial activity in the Aloe. South African Medical Journal. 1987. 81. 984.

Gottshall, R.Y.; Jennings, J.C.; Weller, L.E. et al. Anti-bacterial substances in seed plants active against tubercle bacilli. Am. Rev. Tuberc. 1950. 60. 475-480.

Heggers, J.P.; Winters, W. Aloe and other topical antibacterial agents in wound healing. Aloe Today / Aloecorp. 1993. 8-11. A4

Kahlon, J.B.; Kemp, M.C.; Carpenter, R.H.; McAnalley, B.H.; McDaniel, H.R.; Shannen, W.M. Inhibition of AIDS virus replication by acemannan in vitro. Mol. Biother. 1991. 3. 127-135.

Kahlon, J.B.; Kemp, M.C.; Yawei, N.; Carpenter, R.H.; Shannon, W.M.; McAnalley, B.H. In-vitro evaluation of the synergistic antiviral effects of acemannan in combination with azidothymidine and acyclovir. Mol. Biother. 1991. 3. 214-223.

Levin, H, Harenfratz, R, Fruedman, J, Palevitch, D, Pesl, M., Partial purificaiton and some properties of an antibacterial compound from Aloe Vera. Phytother. Res. 1988. 2(2). 67-69.

Lorenzetti, L.J.; Salisbury, R.; Beal, J.L.; Baldwin, J.N. Bacteriostatic property of Aloe Vera. Journal of Pharmaceutical Science. 1984. 53. 1287.

Mahmoud; Hazem; El-Sibaie; El-Borollosy; El-Kady. Microbiological studies on the Phyllosphere of the desert plant Aloe Vera. Extraction of Anthraquinone-glycosides and Anthraquinone-aglycone from plant leaves, tested as anti-microbial substances against 6 pathogenic and non-pathogenic micro-organisms. 1986. Egypt. J. Microbiol. 21(2) 229-238.

Patel, R.B.; Gandhi, T.P.; Chakravarthy, B.K.; Patel, R J.; Pundarikakshudu, K.; Dhyani, H.K. Antibacterial activity of phenolic and nonphenolic fractions on some Indian medicinal plants. Indian Drugs. 1986. 23(11) 595-597.

Sheets, M.A.; Unger, B.A.; Giggleman, G.F.; Tizard, I.R. Studies of the effect of acemannan on retrovirus infections: clinical stabilization of feline leukemia virus-infected cats. Mol. Biother. 1991. 3. 41-45.

Sims, R.M.; Zimmermann, E.R. Report on effect of Aloe Vera on growth of certain micro-organisms. Baylon College of Dentistry, Dallas Microb Assay Services. 1969. 1. 230-233.

Sims, R.M.; Zimmermann, E.R. Effectiveness of undiluted Aloe 99 gel against Trichomonas Vaginalis, Dallas Microb - Assay Service. Aloe Vera of America Archives, Stabilized Aloe Vera. 1971. 1. 241-242.

Sims, Ruth M.; E.R. Zimmermann Report - The Effect of Aloe Vera on Mycotic Organisms (Fungi) Aloe Vera of America Archives. Stabilized Aloe Vera. 1971. 1. 237-238.

Sims, Ruth M.; E.R. Zimmermann. Effect of Aloe Vera on Herpes Simplex and Herpesvirus (Strain Zoster). Aloe Vera of America Archives. Stabilized Aloe Vera. 1971. 1. 239-240.

Soeda, M.; Osborne, M.; Ome, M.; Kawashima, K. Studies on anti-bacterial and anti-fungal activity of Cape Aloe. Nippon Saikingaku Zasshi 1966. 21. 609-619.

Sydiskis; Owen; Lohr; Rosler; Blomster. Inactivation of Herpes simplex virus by Anthraquinones isolated from plants. J Dental Res. 1989 June. 68. 935.

Sydiskis, R.J.; Owen, D.G.; Lehr, J.L.; Rasler, K.H.; Blomster, R.N. Inactivation of enveloped viruses by anthraquinones extracted from plants. Antimicrob-Agents-Chemother. 1991 Dec. 35(12). 2463-2466.

Syed T.A; Afsal, M.; Ashfa, Q.; Ahmad, S.; Holt, A.N.; Ahmad Ali S.; Ahmad, S.H. Management of genital herpes in men with 0.5% Aloe Vera extract in a hydrophilic cream: a placebo controlled double blind study. J. of Dermatological Treatment. 1997. 8. 99-102.

SECTION IV - USE IN BURNS

The most common nickname attributed to Aloe Vera is "the burn plant". Again, here we find some good research but very few modern clinical studies, despite the fact that Aloe Vera is used quite widely in the USA and even in the UK for general burns and post radiotherapy. Of the current workers, Professor J P Heggars, who is the Head of Research at the Plastic Surgery Department at the University of Galveston, Texas, is perhaps the most celebrated. His work has never been funded by the Aloe industry, unlike several other workers, so is truly independent

Ashley, F.L.; O'Laughlin, B.J.; Peterson, R.; Fernandia, L.; Stein, H.; Schwastz, A.N. The use of Aloe Vera in the treatment of thermal and irradiation burns in laboratory animals and humans. Plastic and Reconstructive Surgery. 1957. 20. 383-396.

Cera, L.M.; Heggers, J.P.; Robson, M.C.; Hagsbrern, W.J. The therapeutic efficacy of Aloe Vera cream dermaide Aloe in thermal injuries 2 cases. J. Am. Anim. Hosp. Assoc. 1980. 16(5). 768-772.

Cera, L.M.; Heggers, J.P.; Hagstrom, W.J.; Robson, M.C. Therapeutic protocol for chemically injured animals and its successful use in an extensively burned rhesus monkey. Journal of the American Animal Hospital Association. 1982. 18. 633-638.

Collins, C.E., M.D. Aloe Vera as a Therapeutic Agent In the treatment of roentgen and radium burns. The Radiological Review and Chicago Medical Recorder. 1935 June. 5(6).

Collins, C.E.; Collins, C. Roentgen dermatitis treated with fresh whole leaf of Aloe Vera. American Journal of Reoentgenology. 1935. 33. 396-397.

Crewe, J.E. Aloes in the treatment of burns and scalds. Minnesota Medicine. 1939. 22. 538-539.

Cutak, L. Aloe Vera as a Remedy for Burns. Missouri Botanical Garden Bulletin. 1937. 25. 169-174.

Loveman, A.B. Leaf of Aloe Vera in Treatment of Roentgen Ray Ulcers. Archives of Dermatology and Syphilology 1937. 36. 838-843.

Lowenthal, L.J.A. Species of Aloe (Other than Aloe Vera) in the Treatment of Roentgen Dermatitis. The Journal of Investigative Dermatology 1949. 12. 295-298.

Lushbaugh, C.C.; Hale, D.B. Experimental acute radiodermatitis following beta radiation. V. histopthological study of the mode of action of therapy with Aloe Vera. Cancer 1953. 6. 690-698.

Mandeville, F.B. Aloe Vera in the treatment of radiation ulcers of mucous membranes. Radiology 1939. 32. 598-599.

Obata, M.; Ibo, S.; Beppu, H.; Fujita, K.; Nagatou, T. Mechanism of anti-inflammatory and antithermal burn action of CPase from Aloe arborescens Miller var natalensis Berger in rats and mice. Phytother. Res. 1993. 7. Special issue. 530-533.

Roberts, D.B.; Travis, E.L. Acemannan containing wound dressing gel reduces radiation-induced skin reactions in C3H mice. Int. J. Radiation Oncol. Biol. Phys. 1995. 32(4) 1047-1052.

Rodriguez-Bigas, M.; Cruz, N.I.; Suarez, A. Comparative evaluation of Aloe Vera in the management of burn wounds in guinea pigs. Plast. Reconstr, Surg. (U.S.) 1988. 81(3). 386-389.

Rowe, T.D. Effect of Fresh Aloe Vera Jelly in the Treatment of Third-Degree Roentgen Reactions on White Rats. Journal of the American Pharmaceutical Association. 1940. 29. 348-350.

Rowe, T.D.; Lovell, B.K.; Parks, L.M. Further observations on the use of Aloe Vera leaf in the treatment of third-degree X-ray reactions. J. of the American Pharmaceutical Assoc. 1991. 30. 266-269.

Ship, A.G. Is topical Aloe Vera plant mucus helpful in burn treatment? J. of the American Medical Assoc. 1977. 238. 1770.

Visuthikasol, V.; Chowchwen, N.; Sukwassarab, Y. Effect of Aloe Vera gel to healing of burn wound - a clinical and histologic study. J. Med. Assoc. Thai. 1993 Aug. 78(8). 703-709.

Visuthikosol, V.; Sukwanarat, Y.; Chowchuen, B.; Sriurairatana, S.; Boonpucknavig, V. Effect of Aloe Vera Gel to healing of burn wound a clinical and histologic study. J. Med. Assoc,. Thai. 1995. 78(8). 403-409. A21

Williams, M.S.; Bink, M.; Loprimzi, C.L.; et. al. Phase III double-blind evaluation of the Aloe Vera gel as a prophylactic agent for radiation induced skin toxicity. Int. J. Radiat. Oncol-Biol-Phys. 1996 Sept. 36(2). 345-349.

Wright, C.S. Aloe Vera in the Treatment of Roentgen Ulcers and Telangiectasis. Journal of the American Medical Association. 1936. 106. 1363-1364.

SECTION V - ANTIDIABETIC EFFECT

Here we have both animal and human studies, the latter only carried out last year in 1996. These two trials in 1996 were placebo controlled and showed that the average (mean) blood glucose level of the patients in the Aloe juice group was significantly reduced from the second week of the study and continued to fall throughout the treatment period. Whereas, there were no changes reported in the placebo group.

Some studies on mice have shown that Aloe causes a rapid decrease in blood sugar as does insulin, but, that the blood glucose level recovers when its administration is discontinued. Beppu et al have demonstrated that there is a glycoprotein in Aloe with a molecular weight of about 50,000 that is a component with a quick hypoglycaemic action, but there are thought to be at least two antidiabetic agents because of differing effects seen when using whole leaf as opposed to gel or pulp. The precise nature of the antidiabetic effect remains unknown. Two animal studies using mice (J.S. Messa 1985) and on rabbits (Roman Ramos 1991) showed little hypoglycaemic activity.

Ajabmoor, M.A. Effects of Aloes on blood glucose levels in normal and alloxan diabetic mice. J. Ethnopharmacology. 1990 Feb. 28(2). 215-220.

Beppu, H.; Nagamura, Y,; Fujita, K. Hypoglycaemic and anti-diabetic effects of Aloe arborescens Miller var. natalensis Berger. International Congress of Phytotherapy. 1991 Oct. Seoul, Korea. 44.

Beppu, H.; Nagamura, Y.; Fujita, K. Hypoglycaemic and anti-diabetic effects in mice of Aloe arborescens Miller var. natalensis Berger. Phytotherapy Research 1993. 7. No special issue. 837-842.

Davis, R.H.; Leitner, M.G.; Russo, J.M. Aloe Vera (A barbadensis). A natural approach for treating wounds, edema, and pain in diabetes. J. Am. Podiatric Med. Assoc. 1988. 78(2). 60-68.

Davis, R.H.; Maro, N.P. Aloe Vera and gibberellin. Anti-inflammatory activity in diabetes. J. Am. Podiatric Med. Assoc. 1989 Jan. 79 (1). 24-26.

Koo, M.W.L Aloe Vera: anti-ulcer and anti-diabetic effects. Phytother Res. 1994. 8(8). 461-464.

Messa, J.S. A study of the crude antidiabetic drugs used in Arabian folk medicine. International Journal of Crude Drug Research. 1985. 23(3). 137-145.

Messa, J.S. A study on the crude antidiabetic drugs used in Arabian folk medicine. Int. J. Crude Drug Res. 1985. 23(3). 137-145. A24

Roman Ramos, R.; Flores Saenz, J.L.; Partida Hermandez, G.; Larca Lemus, A.; Alarcom Aguilar, F. Experimental study of the hypoglycaemic effect of some antidiabetic plants. Arch. Invest. Med.Mex. 1991 Jan-Mar. 22(1) 87-93.

Yongchaiyudia S.; Rungpitakangsi, V.; Bunyapraphatsaran, et al. Antidiabetic activity of Aloe Vera Juice I. Clinical trial in new cases of Diabetes Mellitus. Phytomedicine. 1996. 3(3) 241-243.

Yongchaiyudia S.; Rungpitakangsi, V.; Bunyapraphatsaran, et al. Antidiabetic activity of Aloe Vera Juice II. Clinical trial in new cases of Diabetes Mellitus patients and combination with Glibenclamide Phytomedicine. 1996. 3(3) 245-248.

SECTION VI - CARDIOVASCULAR & LIPID EFFECT

Agarawal combined Aloe Vera and the husk of isabgol (100g and 20g/day respectively) as part of a diet for lunch and dinner in 5000 patients for five years. All had atherosclerotic heart disease and he reported marked decreases in the serum total cholesterol, serum triglyceride, and the fasting and postprandial blood glucose level in diabetic patients. It is interesting that there were no side effects reported amongst this huge trial.

Joshi's animal study has demonstrated that hyperlipidaemic rats fed on Aloe Vera leaves lowered total serum cholesterol, triglycerides, phospholipids and non esterified free fatty acids. Importantly, the high density lipoprotein cholesterol faction (antiatherosclerotic) was elevated.

Agarwal, O.P. Prevention of atheromatous heart diesease. Angiology. 1985. 36(8) 485-492.

Dixit, V.P.; Joshi, S. Effect of Aloe barbadensis and clofibrate on serum lipids in triton induced hyperlipidaemia in presbytis - entellus - entellus monkeys. Indian J. Med. Res. 78 (Sept.) 1983. (Recd. 1984). 417-421.

Joshi, S.; Dixit, V.P. Hypolipidaemic effect of Aloe barbadensis Aloe fraction I in cholesterol fed albino rats I. Lipid and lipoprotein metabolism. Proc. Natl. Acad. Sci. India. SB (Biol. Sci.) 1988. 56(4) 339-342.

Vagi, A.; Shibata, S.; Nishioka, I.; Iwadare, S.; Ishiday, Y. Cardiac stimulant action of constituents of Aloe saponaria. J. of Pharmaceutical Sciences. 1982a. 71. 739-741.

SECTION VII - ANTI-AGEING EFFECT
AND EFFECT ON U.V. LIGHT

Skin ageing is a result of both genetic and environmental factors and one of the most important aspects of the environment is the photo damage caused by UV light. Changes in the dermis affect the overlying skin surface, so with loss of collagen and elastin fibres, giving less support to the epidermis, and with reduced circulatory perfusion, the quality of the skin changes and the wrinkles appear. Associated pigment changes, together with other surface blemishes, produce the typical appearance of old skin. According to Dr Ivan Danhof, true "anti-ageing" actions of a substance requires evidence for the return to normal of the regenerative/degenerative balance exemplified by increased collagen and elastin synthesis. Apart from Vitamin A derivatives and alpha-hydroxy acids, extracts of Aloe Vera can reverse degenerative skin changes and restore the equilibrium in fibre synthesis.

The sun provides the major source of ultra violet radiation and with the possible reduction in stratospheric ozone, the expected increase in ambient UVB radiation is a matter of growing concern. The increase in skin cancers is known to be associated with UV-induced immune suppression. Strickland's studies find that an Aloe Vera extract ameliorated some of the immunosuppressive effects of UV radiation.

Aloe Vera appeared to prevent damage to epidermal dendritic cells but it may be that Aloe exerts its influence later in the chain of immuno-suppressive events or perhaps by inhibiting the formation or release of factors such as TNFα which, amongst others, mediate the T cell immune responses.

Crowell, J.; Nilsenbeck, S.; Penneys, N. Aloe Vera does not affect cutaneous erythema and blood flow following ultraviolet B exposure. Photodermatol 1989 Oct, 6 (5). 237-239.

Danhof I.E. Potential reversal of chronological and photo-ageing of the skin by topical application of natural substances. Phytother Res. 1993. Spec. Issue Proceedings of the International Congress of Phytotherapy, 1991. S53-56.

McKeown, E. Anthraquinones and anthracenic derivatives absorb U.V. light. Cosmetics and Toiletries. 1987 June. 102. 64-65.

Strickland, F.M.; Pelley, R.P.; Kripke, M.L. Prevention of ultraviolet radiation induced suppression of contact and delayed hypersensitivity of Aloe barbadensis gel extract. J. Invest. Dermatol. 1997 Feb. 102(2). 197-204.

Yagi, A.; Kanbara, T.; Morinobu, N. Inhibition of mushroom-tyrosinase by Aloe extract. Planta Medica. 1987. 53(6). 515-517. A10

SECTION VIII - ANTHRAQUINONES

The anthraquinones and their derivatives, otherwise known as the phenolic fraction of the plant, are the source of most of the controversy surrounding products that contain them. Should they be present or not? Are they harmful or not?

Barbaloin in Aloe Vera is a hydroxyanthraquinone, and the majority of evidence does not suggest that this is toxic to man, whereas others containing different chemical sub-groups may be; if taken in large quantities over a long period of time. Even here, the evidence is not conclusive.

Andersen, D.C.; Weber, N.D.; Wood, S.G.; Hughes, B.G.; Murray, B.K.; North, J.A. In vitro virucidal activity of selected anthraquinones and anthraquinone derivatives. Antiviral. Res. 1991. Sep. 16(2). 185-96.

Anton, R.; Haag-Berrurier, M. Therapeutic use of natural Anthraquinones for other than laxative action. Pharmacology 20 (suppl.1) 104-112.

Benigni, R.; Substances with antibiotic action contained in anthraquinonic drugs. Chem. Ab. 1950. 44. 11036.

Brown, J.P. A review of the genetic effects of naturally occurring flavonoids, Anthraquinones and related compounds. Mutat Res. 1980. 75. 243-277.

Capasso, F.; Mascolo N.; Autore, G.; Duraccio, M.R. Effect of Indomethacin on Aloin and 1,8 Dioxianthraquinone-induced Production of Prostaglandins in Rat Isolated Colon. Prostglandins. 1983. 26. 557-562.

Che, Q.M; Akoa, T; Hattori, M; Kobashi, K; Namba, T. Isolation of a human intestinal bacterium capable of transforming barbaloin to aloe-emodin anthrone. Planta Med. 1991 Feb. 57(1). 15-19.

Davis, R.H.; Agnew, P.S.; Shapiro, E. Antiarthritic activity of anthraquinones found in Aloe for podiatric medicine. J. Am. Podiatric Med. Assoc. 1986. 76(2) 61-66.

Davis, R.H.; Leitner, M.G.; Russo, J M; Byrne, M.E. Anti inflammatory activity of Aloe Vera against a spectrum of irritants. J. Am. Podiatric Med. Assoc. (US). 1989 June. 79 (6). 263-276.

Davis; Kabbani; Maro. Aloe Vera and wound healing. Special emphasis to combination with RNA and Vit. C., consideration of part played by Anthraquinones. J. Am. Podiatric Med. Assoc. 1987. 77(4). 165-169.

Fairbairn, J.W.; Simic, S. The Quantitative Conversion of Barbaloin to Aloe-Emodin and its application to the evaluation of Aloes, November 19, 1962 from the Department of Pharmacognosy School of Pharmacy, University of London, Brunswick Square, London, W.C.A. The Journal of Pharmacy and Pharmacology. 1963. 15.

Grimminger, W.; Witthohn, K. Analytics of senna drugs with regard to the toxocological discussions of anthranoids. Pharamacology. 1993 Oct. 47 (Suppl. 1) 98-109.

Heidenmann, A.; Volkner, W.; Mengs, V. Genotoxicity of Aloe Emodin in vitro and in vivo. Mutat Res. 1996 March. 367 (3). 123-133.

Ishii, Y.; Tanizawa, H.; Takino, Y. Studies of Aloe III. Mechanism of cathartic effect. Mechanism of action of Aloe-emodin-9-anthrone, decomposition product of barbaloin in causing significant increase in water content of the rat large intestine. Chem. Pharm. Bull (Tokyo). 1990 Jan. 38(1). 197-200.

Ishii, Y; Tanizawa, H; Takino, Y. Studies of Aloe IV. Mechanism of cathartic effect (3), Biol. Pharm. Bull. 1994 Apr. 17(4) 495-497.

Ishii, Y.; Tanizawa H.; Takino, Y. Studies of Aloe Vera. Mechanism of cathartic effect (4). Biol. Pharm. Bull. 1994 May. 17(5); 651-653.

Koch, A. Investigations of the laxative action of Aloin in the human colon. 41st Annual Congress of the Society of Medicinal Plant Research. Dusseldorf, Germany. 1993 Aug 31-Sept 4. Planta Medica. 59 (Suppl. 7) 1993.

Krumbiegel, G; Schutte, H.V.; Rhein and aloe-Emodin kinetics from senna laxatives in man. Pharmacology. 1993 Oct. 47(Suppl.1) 120-124.

Mahmoud; Hazem; El-Sibaie; El-Borollosy; El-Kady. Microbiological studies on the Phyllosphere of the desert plant Aloe Vera. Extraction of Anthraquinone-glycosides and Anthraquinone-aglycone from plant leaves, tested as anti-microbial substances against 6 pathogenic and non-pathogenic micro-organisms. 1986. Egypt. J. Microbiol. 21(2) 229-238.

Malterud, K.C.; Farbrot, T.L.; Huse, A.E.; Sund, R.B. Antioxidant and radical scavenging effects of anthraquinones and anthrones. Pharmacology. 1993 Oct. 47 (Supp I.1) 77-85.

Mapp, R.K.; McCarthy, T.J. The assessment of purgative principles in Aloes. Planta Medica. 1970. 18. 361-365.

McKeown, E. Anthraquinones and anthracenic derivatives absorb U.V. light. Cosmetics and Toiletries. 1987 June. 102. 64-65.

Odes, H.S.; Madar, Z. A double-blind trial of a Celandin, Aloe Vera and Psyllium laxative preparation in adult patients with constipation. Digestion. 1991. 49. 65-71. A20

Rauwald, H. W; Voetig, R; 7 hydroxyaloin, the leading substance from Aloe Barbadensis in the European Pharmacologica. Arch Pharm. 1982. 315(5). 477-478.

Sendelbach, L.E. A review of the toxicity and carcinogenicity of anthraquinone derivatives. Toxicology. 1989. 57. 227-240. A9

Siegers, C.P.; Siemers, J.; Barettom, G. Sennosides and Aloin do not promote dimethylhydrazine-induced tumours in mice. Pharmacology. 1993 Oct. 47 (Suppl. 7) 205-208.

Siegers, C.P.; von Hertzberg-Lettim, E.; Otte, M.; Schneider, B. Anthranoid laxative abuse - a risk for colorectal cancer? Gut. 1993 Aug. 34(8) 1099-1101.

Sydiskis, R.J.; Owen; Lohr; Rosler; Blomster. Inactivation of Herpes simplex virus by Anthraquinones isolated from plants. J Dental Res. 1989 June. 68. 935.

Sydiskis, R.J.; Owen, D.G.; Lehr, J.L.; Rasler, K.H.; Blomster, R.N. Inactivation of enveloped viruses by anthraquinones extracted from plants. Antimicrob-Agents-Chemother. 1991 Dec. 35(12). 2463-2466.

Westendorf; Marquardt; Poginsky; Dominiak; Schmidt. Genotoxicity of naturally occurring Hydroxyanthraquinones. Evaluation of mutagenicity and cell-transforming activity. Mutat. Res. 1990 Jan. 240(1). 1-12.

Wolfe, D.; Schmutgte, C.; Westendorf, J.; Marquardt, H. Hydroxyanthraquinones as tumour promoters: enhancement of malignant transformation of C3H mouse fibroblasts and growth stimulation of primary rat hepatocytes. Cancer Res. (USA). 1990 Oct. 50(20). 6540-6544.

SECTION IX - GENERAL REVIEWS

Ahmad, S.; Kalhoro, Z.; Kapadia, Z.; Badar, Y. "Aloe" A biologically active and potential medicinal plant. Hamdard. 1993. 36(1). 108-115. A23

Brown, J.P. A review of the genetic effects of naturally occurring flavonoids, anthraquinones and related compounds. Mutat Res. 1980. 75. 243-277.

Bruce, W.G.G. Medicinal Properties in the Aloe. Excelsa 5. 1975. 57-68.

Cole, H.N.; Chen, K.K. Aloe Vera in oriental dermatology. Archives of Dermatology and Syphilology. 1993. 47. 250.

Crewe, J.E.. The External Use of Aloes. Minnesota Medicine. 1937. 20. 670-673.

Danhof, I.E. Aloe in cosmetics - does it do anything? Cosmet Toilet. 1987. 102. 62-63.

Davis, R.N. Biological activity of Aloe Vera. Seigen, Oele, Fette, Wachse (Germany). 1993 Sept. 119. 646-649.

Fischer, J.M. Medical Use of Aloe Products. US Pharm. 1982 Aug. 7. 37-45.

Flagg, J. Aloe Vera Gel in Dermatological Preparations. Am Perfum Cosmet. 1959. 74. 27-29.

Gjerstad, G.; Riner, T.D. Current status of Aloe as a cure-all. American Journal of Pharmacy. 1968. 140. 58-64.

Goldberg, H.C. The Aloe Vera Plant. Archives of Dermatology and Syphilology. 1944. 49. 46.

Grindlay, D. Aloe Vera. The Garden. Journal of the Royal Horticultural Society. 1985. 110, 534-535.

Grindlay, D. Medical use of Aloe Vera. General Practitioner (London). 1985 June.

Grindlay, D., Reynolds, T.. The Aloe Vera Phenomenon: A Review of the Properties and Modern Uses of the Leaf Parenchyma Gel. J. Ethnopharmacol. 1986. 16. 117-151.

Haller, J.S. A drug for all seasons, medical and pharmacological history of Aloe. Bull. N.Y. Acad. Med. 1990. 66(6). 647-659. A14

Harendal, B.E. Whole leaf Aloe Vera: almost a panacea. Health Conscious. 1992. 13(1). 14-17.

Harrison, J. Aloe in Dentistry. Health Conscious. 1992. 13 (1) 19-24.

Klein, AD, Penneys, NS. Aloe Vera. J. of Am. Ac. Derm. 1988. 18(4,1) 714-720.

Leung, A. Aloe Vera update: new form questions integrity of old. Drug Cosmet Ind. 1985 Sept. 137-42, 44-46.

Marshall, J.M. Aloe Vera Gel: what is the evidence? The Pharmaceutical Journal. 1990. 360-362.

McKeown, E. Aloe Vera. Cosmetics & Toiletries. 1987. 102. 64-65.

Natow, A.J. Aloe Vera fiction or fact. Cutis. 1986. 37(2). 106-108.

Reynolds, T. The compounds in Aloe leaf exudates: a review. Botanical Journal of the Linnaean Society. 1985. 90. 157-177.

Robson, M.C.; Heggers, J.P.; Hagstrom. W.J. Myth, magic, witchcraft or fact? Aloe Vera revisited. Journal of Burn Care and Rehabilitation. 1982. 3. 157-163.

Spoerke, D.G.; Ekims, B.R. Aloe Vera - fact or quackery (medicinal plants). Veterinary and Human Toxicology. 1980. 22. 418-429.

Tchou, M.T. Aloe Vera (Jelly Leeks). Archives of Dermatology and Syphilology. 1943. 47. 249.

Tolbert, T.L. Aloe Vera: past, present and future. Seigen, Oele, Fette, Wachse (Germany). 1997 Jan. 120. 14-18.

Tyler, V. Aloe. The Honest Herbal. 25-28. A18

Vogler, B.K.; Ernst, E. Aloe Vera: A systematic review of its clinical effectiveness. British Journal of General Practice 1999, 49, 823-828.

SECTION X - WOUND HEALING

The paper by J.E. Fulton in 1990 on the effects of Aloe Vera on post-dermabrasion wound healing was the paper that inspired me to carry out my own research into Aloe Vera. I was intrigued by its conclusion - "the reasons for the accelerated wound healing are unknown"!

Virtually all papers show positive results demonstrating Aloe's wound healing potential as it plays a part in this complex system. However, there is one important paper that showed a delay in wound healing, that of Schmidt and Greenspoon Published in 1991. They applied topical Aloe Vera to post Caesarian wounds with negative results. I first wonder whether the change in hormonal status of these patients interferes with the action of Aloe Vera.

Barnes, T.C. The healing action of extracts of Aloe Vera leaf on abrasions of human skin. American Journal of Botany. 1997. 39. S97.

Bishop, J.B.; Philips, L.G.; Musbore, T.A. et. al. A prospective randomised evaluation - blinded trial of two potential wound-healing agents for the treatment of venous stasis ulcers. J. Vasc. Surg. 1992. 16. 251-257.

Bradshaw, T.W. Aloe Vera: its influence on the physiology of wound healing and inflammation. J. Brit. Pod. Med. 1996. 51(2). 25-29.

Davis R.H.; Didonato J.J.; Hartman G.M.; Haas R.C. Anti-Inflammatory and wound healing activity of a growth substance in Aloe Vera. J. Am. Podiatric Med. Assoc. 1984 Feb. 84:.

Davis R.H.; Kabbani J.M.; Maro, N.P. Wound Healing. J. Am. Podiatric Med. Assoc. 1987 April. 77. 4.

Davis, R.H.; Leitner, M.G.; Russo, J.M.; Byrne, M.E. Wound healing, oral and topical activity of Aloe Vera. J. Am. Podiatric Med. Assoc. 1989 Nov, 79(11). 559-562.

Davis, R.H.; Parker, W.L.; Samson, R.T.; Murdoch, D.S. Isolation of a stimulatory system in aloe extract. J. Am. Podiatric Med. Soc. 1991 Sept. 81(9) 473-477.

Davis, R.H. Influence of Aloe on inflammation and wound healing. International Congress of Phytotherapy. 1991 Oct. Seoul, Korea. 29.

Davis, R.H.; Didonato, J.J.; Hartman, G.M.; Haas, R.C. Anti-inflammatory and wound healing activity of a growth substance in Aloe Vera. J. Am. Podiatric. Med. Assoc. 1994 Feb. 84(2). 77-81.

Davis, R.H.; Leitner, M.G.; Russo, J.M. Aloe Vera (A barbadensis). A natural approach for treating wounds, edema, and pain in diabetes. J. Am. Podiatric Med. Assoc. 1988. 78(2). 60-68.

Davis; Kabbani; Maro. Aloe Vera and wound healing. Special emphasis to combination with RNA and Vit. C., consideration of part played by Anthraquinones. J. Am. Podiatric Med. Assoc. 1987. 77(4). 165-169.

El Zawahry, M.; Hegarty, M.R.; Helal, M. Use of Aloe in treating leg ulcers and dermatoses. International J. of Dermatology. 1973. 12. 68-73.

Fulton, J.E. The stimulation of postdermabrasion wound healing with stabilised Aloe Vera gel-polyethylene oxide dressing. J. Dermatol Surg. Oncol. 1990 May. 16(5). 460-467.

Heggers, J.P.; Kucukcelebi, A.; Listengarten, D.; Stabenau, J.; Ko, F.; Broemeliing, L.D.; Robson, M.C.; Winters, W.D. Beneficial effect of Aloe on wound healing in an excisional wound model. J. of Alternative and Complementary Medicine. 1966. 2(2). 271-277.

Heggers, J.P.; Robson, M.C. Beneficial effects of Aloe in wound healing. International Congress of Phytotherapy. 1991 Oct. Seoul, Korea. 27.

Heggers, J.P.; Pelley, R.P.; Robson, M.C. Beneficial effects of Aloe in wound healing. Phytother. Res. 1993. 7. No special issue. S48-52.

Heggers, J.P.; Winters, W. Aloe and other topical antibacterial agents in wound healing. Aloe Today / Aloecorp. 1993. 8-11. A4

Heggers, J.P.; Haussam, E.; Garfield, R. et. al. Effect of the combination of Aloe Vera, nitroglycerin and L-NAME on wound healing in the rat excisional model. J. of Alternative and Complementary Medicine. 1997. 3(2). 149-153.

Kaufman, T.; Kalderom, N.; Ullmann, Y.; Berger, J. Aloe Vera gel hindered wound healing of experimental second-degree burns; a quantitative controlled study. J. Burn Care Rehabil. 1988 Mar-Apr. 9(2), 156-159.

Knight, J.H.; Stevens, E. Anti-inflammatory and healing properties of Aloe barbadensis. International Congress of Phytotherapy 1991 Oct. Seoul, Korea. 31.

Martinet, C.; Guardarama, I.; Arcas, E. Preclinical and clinical evaluation of the cicatrizant effects of Aloe Barbadensis. Revista Farmaceutica (Argentina). 1993. 135. 101-106.

McCauley, R.L.; Heggers, J.P.; Robson, M.C. Frostbite - methods to minimise tissue loss. Frostbite. 1990. 88(8). 72-77.

Miller, M.B.; Koltai, P.J. Treatment of experimental frostbite with pentoxifylline and Aloe Vera cream. Arch. Otolaringol Head Neck Surg. 1995 June. 121(6). 678-680.

Morsy, E.M.; Ovaniviski, H. Evaluating the healing characteristics of the exuded mucilage from Aloe Barbadensis Miller. J. of Technical Information on botanical and animal active ingredients for the cosmetic, perfumery and flavour industries. Special issue on Aloe Vera. 1993 June. 1. 1-80.

Plemens, J.M.; Rees, T.D.; Binnie, W.H.. et al. Evaluation of acemannan in the treatment of recurrent aphthous stomatitis. Wounds. 1994. 6(2) 40-45.

Schmidt, J.M.; Greenspoon, J.S. Aloe Vera dermal wound gel is associated with a delay in wound healing. Obstet, Gynaecol (U.S.) 1991 July. 78(1). 115-117.

Sumano Lopez, H.; Camberros, L.B.; Ocampo, A.A.; De Lepez, H.S. Comparative evaluation of a mixture of propolis and Aloe Vera with commercial wound healing products. Veterimarcia Mexico. 1989. 20(4). 408-414.

Swain, S.F.; Riddell, K.P.; McGuire, J.A. Effects of topical medications on the healing of open pad wounds in dogs. J. of the American Animal Hosp. Assoc. 1992. 28(6). 499-502.

Thomlinson, R.H. Kitchen Remedy for Necrotic Malignant Breast Ulcers. Lancet. 1980. 2: 707.

Tizard, I.R.; Maxwell, B.; Kemp, M.C. et. al. Accelerated wound healing induced by macrophage stimulants in rats: a genetically controlled phenomenon. Wound Repair and regeneration. 1993. 1. 130.

Udupa, S.L.; Udupa, A.L.; Kulkarmi, D.R. Anti-inflammatory and wound healing properties of Aloe Vera. Fitoterapia. 1994. 65(2). 141-145.

Watcher, M.A.; Wheeland, R.G. The role of topical agents in the healing of full thickness wounds. J. Dermatol. Surg. Oncol. 1989 Nov. 15(11). 1188-1195.

SECTION XI - CONTENTS, CHEMISTRY AND BIOLOGICAL ACTIVITIES

There are several papers in this group showing the widespread interest in the plant's chemistry. Not all researchers come up with the same findings as would be expected because of the variety of specimens used. The constituents of an Aloe Vera plant will vary depending on (i) its botanical variety, (ii) its age, (iii) the type of soil in which it was grown, (iv) the amount of sunshine to which it was subjected, and (v) the season in which it was harvested.

Beppu, H.; Fujita, K. Isolation and the pharmacological activities of the effective compounds Aloe arborescens Miller var Natalensis Berger. International Congress of Phytotherapy. 1991 Oct. Seoul, Korea. 37.

Danhof, I.E.; McAnally, B.H. Stabilized Aloe Vera. 1983.

Davenport, L. Pharmacists and the silent healer Aloe Vera. Texas Pharmacy. 1994 July. 113. 18-19.

Davis, R.H.; Leitner, M.G.; Russo, J.M.; Maro, N.P. Biological activity of Aloe Vera. Med. Sci. Res. 1987. 15(5). 235-236.

Davis, R.N. Biological activity of Aloe Vera. Siegen, Oele, Fette, Wachse (Germany). 1993 Sept. 119. 646-649.

Fujita, K.; Teradoura, R.; Nagatsu, T. Bradykinase activity of Aloe extract. Biochemical Pharmacology. 1976. 25. 205.

Fujita, K.; Ito, S.; Teradaira, R.; Beppu, H. Properties of carboxypeptidase from Aloe. Biochemical Pharmacology. 1979. 28. 1261-1262.

Gerloff, D.R. Study of the organoleptic properties of the exuded mucilage from the Aloe barbadensis leaves. Erde International. J of Technical Information on botanical and animal active ingredients for the cosmetic, perfumery and flavour industries. Special issue on Aloe Vera. 1993 April-June. 1(1) 1-80.

Gjerstad, G. Chemical studies of Aloe Vera Juice I. Amino Acid Analysis. Advancing Frontiers of Plant Sciences. 1971. 28. 311-315.

Gouda, D.C.; Neelisiddaiah, B; Amjaneyalu, Y.V. Structural studies of polysaccharides from Aloe Vera. Carbohydrate Research. 1979. 72. 201-205.

Henry, C.R. Identification and standardisation of Aloe Vera as a biological active ingredient for topical and internal products International Congress of Phytotherapy. 1991 Oct. Seoul, Korea. 57.

Hirata, T.; Suga, T. Biologically active constituents of leaves and roots of Aloe arborescens var natalensis. Zeitschript pur Naturforschung. 1977. 32. 731-734.

Hranisavijevic-Jakovijevic, M.; Miijkovic-Stojanovic, J. Structural Study of an Acidic Polysaccharide Isolated from Aloe Arborescens Mill. 1 Periodate Oxidation and Partial Acid Hydrolysis. Glasnik Hemiskog Drustva. Beograd. 1981. 46. 269-273.

Ibo, S; Teradaira, R.; Beppu, H; Obata, M.; Nagatsu, T.; Fujita, K. Properties and pharmacological activity of carboxypeptidase in Aloe arborescens Miller var. natalensis Berger. International Congress of Phytotherapy. 1991 Oct. Seoul, Korea. 39.

Ibo, S; Teradaira, R; Beppu, H; Obata. M.; Fijita, K; Nagabsu, T. Biochemical properties of carboxypeptidase from Aloe arborescens Miller var. natalensis Berger. Phytotherapy Research. 1993. 7. No special issue. S26-29.

Imanishi, Keni Chi. Aloctin A, an active substance of Aloe arborescens as an immunomodulator. International Congress of Phytotherapy. 1991 Oct. Seoul, Korea 34.

Imanishi, Kimichi, Aloctin, A. An active substance of Aloe arborescens as an immunomodulator. Phytother. Res. (1993) 7 (Spec. Issue). Proceedings of the International Congress of Phytotherapy. 1991. S20-22.

Ishii, Y.; Tanizawa, H.; Takino, Y. Studies of Aloe III. Mechanism of cathartic effect. Mechanism of action of Aloe-emodin-9-anthrone, decomposition product of barbaloin in causing significant increase in water content of the rat large intestine. Chem. Pharm. Bull (Tokyo). 1990 Jan. 38(1). 197-200.

Ishii, Y; Tanizawa, H; Takino, Y. Studies of Aloe IV. Mechanism of cathartic effect (3), Biol. Pharm. Bull. 1994 Apr. 17(4) 495-497.

Ishii, Y.; Tanizawa H.; Takino, Y. Studies of Aloe Vera. Mechanism of cathartic effect (4). Biol. Pharm. Bull. 1994 May. 17(5); 651-653.

Ibo, S.; Teradaira, R.; Beppu, H.; Obata, M.; Fujita, K.; Nagatsu, T. Biochemical properties of Carboxypeptidase from Aloe arborescens Miller var. natalensis Berger. Phytother. Res. 1993. 7. S26-29.

Koch, A. Investigations of the laxative action of Aloin in the human colon. 41st Annual Congress of the Society of Medicinal Plant Research. Dusseldorf, Germany. 1993 Aug 31-Sept 4. Planta Medica. 59 (Suppl. 7) 1993.

Malterud, K.C.; Farbrot, T.L.; Huse, A.E.; Sund, R.B. Antioxidant and radical scavenging effects of anthraquinones and anthrones. Pharmacology. 1993 Oct. 47 (Supp I.1) 77-85.

Mandal, G.; Das, A. Structure of the gluco-mannan isolated from the leaves of Aloe Barbadensis Miller. Carbohydrate Research. 1980. 87. 249-256.

Mandal, G.; Ghash, R.; Das, A. Characterisation of polysaccharides of Aloe Barbadensis Miller. Part III. Structure of acidic oligosaccharide. Indian Journal of Chemistry. 1993. 22B. 890-893.

Mapp, R.K.; McCarthy, T.J. The assessment of purgative principles in Aloes. Planta Medica. 1970. 18. 361-365.

Nouri, Y. Mary, Christensen, Bernard, and Beals, Jack 1. The Effect of Some Selected Surface-Active Agents on the Extraction of Cape Aloe. Journal of the American Pharmaceutical Association. 1956. 45 (6).

Parry, O; Matambo, C. Some pharmacological actions of Aloe extracts and Cassia abbreviata on rats and mice. Cent. Afr. J. Med. 1992 Oct. 38(1C). 409-414.

Pierce, R.F. Comparison between the nutritional contents of the Aloe gel form conventionally and hydroponically grown plants. Erde International Journal of Technical Information on botanical and animal active ingredients for the cosmetic, perfumery and flavour industries. Special issue on Aloe Vera. 1993 Apr.-June. 1(1). 1-80.

Reynolds, T. Observations on the phytochemistry of the Aloe leaf-exudate compounds. Botanical Journal of the Linnean Society. 1985. 90. 179-199.

Reynolds, T. The compounds in Aloe leaf exudates: a review. Botanical Journal of the Linnaean Society. 1985. 90. 157-177.

Roboz, E.; Haagen-Smit, A.J. A Mucilage from Aloe Vera. Journal of the American Chemical Society. 1948. 70. 3248-3249.

Rowe, T.D.; Parks, L.M. Phytochemical Study of Aloe Vera Leaf. Journal of the American Pharmaceutical Association. 1941. 30. 262-266.

Rubel, B.L. Possible mechanisms of the healing actions of Aloe gel. Cosmetics and Toiletries. 1983. 98. 109-119.

Saga, T.; Hirata, T. The efficacy of the Aloe plants: chemical constituents and biological activities. Cosmet. Toiletries. 1983. 98. 105-108.

Saito; Hiroko. Purification of active substances of Aloe arborescens Miller and their biological and pharmacological activity. Phytother. Res. 1993. 7. Spec. Issue, Proceedings of the International Congress of Phytotherapy. 1991. S17-19.

Shahmaz A.; Kalhoro, M.A.; Kapadia, Z.; Yasmeem, B. "Aloe", a biologically active and potential medicinal plant. Hamdard Medicus. 1993. 36(1). 108-115.

Shelton, M.S. Aloe Vera, Its Chemical and Therapeutical Properties. International Journal of Dermatology. 1991. 30. 679-683.

Wang, Y.T; Strong, K. J. Monitoring physical and chemical properties of freshly harvested field-grown Aloe Vera leaves. A preliminary report. Phytother. Res. (1993) 7. Spec. Issue. Proceedings of the International Congress of Phytotherapy. 1991. S1-4.

Yagi, A.; Makino, K.; Nishioka, I.; Kuchino, Y. Aloe Mannan, Polysaccharide, from Aloe Arborescens var. Natalensis. Planta Medica. 1977. 31. 17-20.

Yamaguchi, I; Mega, N; Sanada, H. Components of the gel of Aloe Vera (L.) burn. f. Biosci. Biotechnol. Biochem. 1993 Aug. 57(8). 1350-1352.

Yamamoto, M.; Sugiyama, K.; Yokota, M.; Maeda, Y.; Inaoka, Y. Study of possible pharmacological actions of Aloe Barbadensis Miller on mouse, hamster and human skin. Aloenin - major constituent of Aloe - effect of sebaceous gland size, hair growth and damaged skin. Japanese Journal of Toxicology and Environmental Health. 1993. 39(5). 404-414.

SECTION XII - GASTROINTESTINAL EFFECTS

Here there is only one paper looking at the effect of orally consumed Aloe Vera gel on normal humans and this trial carried out by Dr Jeffrey Bland, although important, is really too small, as he only used ten volunteers. There needs to be a lot more work here on Aloe's effect on disordered gastro-intestinal tracts, especially in the areas of IBS and chronic inflammatory bowel disease where anecdotal evidence for its success abounds.

Bland, J. Effect of orally consumed Aloe Vera juice on gastrointestinal function in normal humans. Linus Pauling Institute of Science & Medicine Palo Alto, C.A. Prevention Magazine. 1985.

Blitz, J.J.; Smith, J.W.; Gerard, J.R. Aloe Vera Gel in peptic ulcer therapy: preliminary report. Journal of the American Osteopathic Association. 1963. 62. 731-735.

Che, Q.M; Akoa, T; Hattori, M; Kobashi, K; Namba, T. Isolation of a human intestinal bacterium capable of transforming barbaloin to aloe-emodin anthrone. Planta Med. 1991 Feb. 57(1). 15-19.

Heggers, J.P.; Nealon, W.; Pelley, R.P. The effect of oral administration of Aloe gel extracts upon the induction of cysteamine-induced gastric and duodenal ulcers in the male sprague Dawley rat. International Congress of Phytotherapy. 1991 Oct. Seoul, Korea. 52.

Koo, M.W.L Aloe Vera: anti-ulcer and anti-diabetic effects. Phytother Res. 1994. 8(8). 461-464.

Parman, N.S.; Tario, M.; Al-Yahya, M.A.; Ageel, A.M.; Al-Said, M.S. Evaluation of Aloe Vera leaf exudate and gel for gastric and duodenal anti-ulcer activity. Fitoterapia 57(5). 1986 (recd. 1987). 380-383.

Teradaira, R.; Shimzato, M.; Beppu, H.; Fujita, K. Antigastric ulcer effects in rats of Aloe arborescens Miller var. natalensis Berger extract. Phytother. Res. 1993. 7 (No special issue). 534-536.

SECTION XIII - IMMUNOMODULATION

This is really the story of the long chain polysaccharide, Acemannan, and for anyone interested in pursuing this aspect of Aloe the entire research evidence gathered by Carrington Laboratories in the USA, leading to the development of their product "Carrisyn" is available. The document produced in July 1992 is entitled "Pharmacologic effects and mechanisms of action of Acemannan", and is available from Carrington Laboratories, 2001 Walnut Hill Lane, Irving, Texas 75038.

Carpenter, R H.; Yates, K.M.; Busbee, D.; King, G.; Tizard, I.; McAnalley, B. Clinical applications of a biological response modifier (acemannan) in veterinary clinical medicine. International Congress of Phytotherapy. 1991 Oct. Seoul, Korea 62.

Clumeck, N.; Hermans, P. Antiviral drugs other than zidovudine and immunomodulating therapies in human immunodeficiency virus infection. The Am. J. of Med. 1988. 85 (Suppl. 2A) 165-170.

Green P. Aloe Vera extracts in equine clinical practice. Veterinary Times. 1996 Sept. 26(9) 16.

Hahn, Dug-Ryong. A national polysaccharide having activity on the reticuloendothelial system from Aloe Vera exudate. International Congress of Phytotherapy. 1991 Oct. Seoul, Korea.

Harris, C.; Pierce, K.; King, G.; Yates, K.M.; Hall, J.; Tizard, I. Efficacy of acemannan in treatment of canine and feline spontaneous neoplasms. Mol. Biother. 1991. 3. 207-213.

Hart, L.A.; van Emckevort, P.H; van Dijk, H; Faat, R; de Silva, K.T.; Labodie, R.P. Two functionally and chemically distinct immunomodulatory compounds in the gel of Aloe Vera . J. Ethnopharmacol. 1988 May-Jun. 23(1). 61-71.

Imanishi, Keni Chi. Aloctin A, an active substance of Aloe arborescens as an immunomodulator. International Congress of Phytotherapy. 1991 Oct. Seoul, Korea 34.

Imanishi, Kimichi, Aloctin, A. An active substance of Aloe arborescens as an immunomodulator. Phytother. Res. (1993) 7 (Spec. Issue). Proceedings of the International Congress of Phytotherapy. 1991. S20-22.

Kahlon, J.B.; Kemp, M.C.; Yawei, N.; Carpenter, R.H.; Shannon, W.M.; McAnalley, B.H. In-vitro evaluation of the synergistic antiviral effects of acemannan in combination with azidothymidine and acyclovir. Mol. Biother. 1991. 3. 214-223.

Karaca, K.; Sharma, J.M.; Nordgren, R. Nitric oxide production by chicken macrophages activated by acemannan, a complex carbohydrate extracted from Aloe Vera. International Journal of Immunopharmacology. 1993. 17(3). 183-188.

Marshall, G.D.; Druck, J.P. In vitro stimulation of NK activity by acemannan (ACM). J. Immunol. 1993. 150. 1381.

Marshall, G.D.; Gibbons, A.S.; Parnell, L.S. Human cytokines induced by acemannan. J. Allergy Clin. Immunol. 1993. 91. 295.

McAnalley, B.H.; Carpenter, R.H.; McDaniel, H.R. Uses of acemannan of other Aloe products in the treatment of diseases requiring intervention of the immune system for cure. Carrington Laboratories Inc. USA. PCT Int. Appl. 115. CODEN. PIXXD2.

McDaniel, H.R.; McAnalley, B.H. Evaluation of polymannoacetate (Carrisyn) in the treatment of AIDS. Clin. Res. 1987. 35. 483A.

McDaniel, H.R.; Perkins, S.; McAnalley, B.N. A clinical pilot study using Carrisyn TM in the treatment of acquired immunodeficiency syndrome (AIDS). Ass. J. Clin. Pathol. 1987. 88-534.

Peng, S.Y.; Norman, J.; Curtim, G.; Corrier, D.; McDaniel, H.R.; Busbee, D. Decreased mortality of Norman murine sarcoma in mice treated with the immunomodulator, acemannan. Mol. Biother. 1991. 3. 79-87.

Rakatovao, L.H.; LeDeaut, J.Y. Mise en Evidence et Etude des Proprietes Immunostimulantes d;un extrait isole et partiellement purifie a partir d'Aloe Vahombe. Archives de L'Institut Pasteur de Madagascar. 1979. 47. 9-39.

Sheets, M.A.; Unger, B.A.; Giggleman, G.F.; Tizard, I.R. Studies of the effect of acemannan on retrovirus infections: clinical stabilization of feline leukemia virus-infected cats. Mol. Biother. 1991. 3. 41-45.

Tizard, I.; Carpenter, R.H.; Kemp, M. Immuno-regulatory effects of a cytokine release enhancer (acemannan). International Congress of Phytotherapy 1991 Oct Seoul, Korea 68.

Winters; Wendell. Immunoreactive lectins in leaf gel from Aloe Barnadensis Miller. Phytother. Res. 1993. 7. Spec. Issue, Proceedings of the International Congress of Phytotherapy. 1991. S23-25.

Womble, D.; Helderman, J.H. The impact of acemannan on the generation and function of cytotoxic T-lymphocytes. Immunopharmacol Immunotoxicol. 1992. 14. 63-77.

SECTION XIV - MISCELLANEOUS

Although not specifically on Aloe Vera, I recommend the reading of Sharma's article on Phytochemical Synergism in "Alternative therapies in clinical practice". This concept, foreign to allopathic medicine, underpins the action of Aloe Vera.

Anderson, B.C.. Aloe Vera Juice: A veterinary predicament. The Compendium on Continuing Education for the Practising Veterinarian 5. 1983. S364-S368.

Ashleye, A.D. Applying heat during processing the commercial Aloe Vera gel. Erde International Journal of Technical Information on botanical and animal active ingredients for the cosmetic, perfumery and flavour industries. Special issue on Aloe Vera. 1993 Apr.-June. 1 (1). 1-80.

Carpenter, R H.; Yates, K.M.; Busbee, D.; King, G.; Tizard, I.; McAnalley, B. Clinical applications of a biological response modifier (acemannan) in veterinary clinical medicine. International Congress of Phytotherapy. 1991 Oct. Seoul, Korea 62.

Fine, A.F.; Brown, S. Cultivation and Clinical Application of Aloe Vera Leaf. Radiology. 1938. 31. 735-736.

Fujita, K.; Suzuki, I.; Ochiai, J.; Shinpo, J.; Inaue, S and Saito, H. Specific reaction of Aloe extract with serum proteins of various animals. Experientia. 1978. 39. 523-524.

Garnick, J.; Hanes, P.J.; Hardim, J.; Thompson, W. Changes in root sensitivity with toothpastes containing Aloe Vera and allantoin. Archives of Oral Biology. 1994. 39 (Suppl.) 132S.

Green P. Aloe Vera extracts in equine clinical practice. Veterinary Times. 1996 Sept. 26(9) 16.

Harrison, J. Aloe in Dentistry. Health Conscious. 1992. 13 (1) 19-24. Kawai, K.; Beppu, H.; Koike, T.; Fujita, K.; Marunouchi, T. Tissue culture of Aloe arborescens Miller var. natalensis Berger. Phytother. Res. 1993. 7. S5-10.

Klabim, G. Processing of Aloe Vera leaves for whole-leaf products; revealing the secrets of the producers. Health Conscious. 1992. 13(1). 47-48.

Meadows, T.P. Aloe as a humectant in new skin preparations. Cosmetics and Toiletries. 1980. 95. 51-56.

Nath, D.; Sethi, N.; Singh, R.K.; Jaim, A.K. Commonly used Indian abortifacient plants with special reference to their teratologic effects in rats. J. of Ethnopharmacol. 38(2). 147-159.

Newton, L.E. In Defence of the name Aloe Vera. The Cactus and Succulent Journal of Great Britain. 1979. 41. 29-30.

Northway, R.B. Experimental use of Aloe Vera extract in clinical practice. Veterinary Medicine/Small Animal Clinician. 1975. 70. 89.

Oh, You-Jin; Heng, Jin-Tai; et al. Effects of Aloe Vera and Aloe arborescens mixture on cirrhosis patients. International Congress of Phytotherapy. 1991 Oct. Seoul, Korea. 42.

OSW, C.S.; Bokadia, M.M. The effect of extracts of Aloe barbadensis M.11 leaves on the fertility of female rats. Indian Drugs. 1979. 16(6). Mar. 125-127.

Parry, O.; Wenyika, J. The uterine relaxant effect of Aloe. Chapandi: Fitoterapia 1994. 65(3). 253-259.

Pelley, R.P.; Wang, Y.T.; Waller, T.A. Current status of quality control of Aloe Barbadensis extracts. SOFW Journal. 1993. 119. 255-268.

Sharma, H.M. Phytochemical synergism: beyond the active ingredient model. Alternative Therapies in Clinical Practice. 1997. 4(3). 91-96.

Sturm, P.G.; Hayes, S.M. Aloe Vera in Dentistry. J Bergen Cty. Dent. Soc. 1989 May. SO(8). 11-14.

Syed T.A.; Ahmad Ashfares; Holt, A.H.; Ahmad Seyed A.; Ahmad S.H.; Afzal M. Management of psoriasis with Aloe Vera cream tropical medicine and international health. 1996. 1(4) 505-509.

Yamoto, W.W. Formulating beverage products from the stabilised Aloe gel. Erde International. Journal of Technical Information on botanical and animal active ingredients for the cosmetic, perfumery and flavour industries. Special issue on Aloe Vera. 1993 April-June. 1 (1) 1-80.

Yaron; Amima. Characteristics of Aloe Vera gel before and after autodegradation, and stabilisation of the natural fresh gel. Phytother. Res. 1993. 7. Spec. Issue, Proceedings of the International Congress of Phytotherapy. 1991. S11-13.

SECTION XV - SIDE EFFECTS AND TOXICOLOGY

Aloe Vera gel itself produces virtually no side effects and is extremely safe! Occasionally a discoid form of eczema has been reported after oral use.

Dominguert-Soto, L. Photodermatitis to Aloe Vera (letter, comment). Int. J. Dermatol. 1992 May. 31(5). 372.

Heidenmann, A.; Volkner, W.; Mengs, V. Genotoxicity of Aloe Emodin in vitro and in vivo. Mutat Res. 1996 March. 367 (3). 123-133.

Morrow, D.M.; Rapaport, M.J.; Strick, R.A. Hypersensitivity to Aloe. Arch Dermatol. 1980. 116(9). 1064-1065.

Sendelbach, L.E. A review of the toxicity and carcinogenicity of anthraquinone derivatives. Toxicology. 1989. 57. 227-240. A9

Siegers, C.P.; von Hertzberg-Lettim, E.; Otte, M.; Schneider, B. Anthranoid laxative abuse - a risk for colorectal cancer? Gut. 1993 Aug. 34(8) 1099-1101.

Westendorf; Marquardt; Poginsky; Dominiak; Schmidt. Genotoxicity of naturally occurring Hydroxyanthraquinones. Evaluation of mutagenicity and cell-transforming activity. Mutat. Res. 1990 Jan. 240(1). 1-12.

NOTES

NOTES

NOTES

NOTES

NOTES

NOTES